ANXIETY
IN RELATIONSHIP

How to Eliminate Negative Thinking, Jealousy, Attachment and Overcome Couple Conflicts. Insecurity and Fear of Abandonment Often Cause Irreparable Damage Without Therapy, Couples Therapy, Skills

Teresa Williams Dr Miller Scarlett

© Copyright 2020 by Teresa Williams Dr Miller Scarlett

All rights reserved.

The work contained herein has been produced with the intent to provide relevant knowledge and information on the topic on the topic described in the title for entertainment purposes only. While the author has gone to every extent to furnish up to date and true information, no claims can be made as to its accuracy or validity as the author has made no claims to be an expert on this topic. Notwithstanding, the reader is asked to do their own research and consult any subject matter experts they deem necessary to ensure the quality and accuracy of the material presented herein.

This statement is legally binding as deemed by the Committee of Publishers Association and the American Bar Association for the territory of the United States. Other jurisdictions may apply their own legal statutes. Any reproduction, transmission or copying of this material contained in this work without the express written consent of the copyright holder shall be deemed as a copyright violation as per the current legislation in force on the date of publishing and subsequent time thereafter. All additional works derived from this material may be claimed by the holder of this copyright.

The data, depictions, events, descriptions and all other information forthwith are considered to be true, fair and accurate unless the work is expressly described as a work of fiction. Regardless of the nature of this work, the Publisher is exempt from any responsibility of actions taken by the reader in conjunction with this work. The Publisher acknowledges that the reader acts of their own accord and releases the author and Publisher of any responsibility for the observance of tips, advice, counsel, strategies and techniques that may be offered in this volume.

TABLE OF CONTENTS

Introduction 1

Chapter 1: Understanding The Reasons Behind The Feelings Of Insecurity, Anxiety, And Attachment 3

    Common Signs Of Relationship Anxiety 5

    Breeding Anxious Feelings And Thoughts.................... 12

    Why Do You Feel Insecure, Attached, And Anxious In A Relationship? 15

    Signs Related To Insecure Attachment........................ 20

        Very Demanding 20

        Jealousy Or Doubt... 21

        Enthusiastic Dependency 21

        Anger Issues.. 21

Chapter 2: Reasons Behind Irrational Behaviors Resulting From Anxiety 22

    Irrational Behaviors Resulting From Anxiety............... 24

        Unwarranted Irritability 25

        Compulsive Behavior 26

        Excessive Worrying 26

        Physical Aggression.. 27

        Moping 28

    Need For Understanding Your Partner 28

    Lack Of Understanding – The Prime Reason Behind Relationship Failures... 32

    Control Your Body Language And Manners 34

    Make Communication A Daily Habit 35

    Not Forcing Your Partner To Change 35

    Choosing The Perfect Time... 36

Practical Ways Of Getting To Know Your Partner In A Better Way 36

   Spending Time With Their Friends 36
   Plan A Vacation 37
   Sharing Hobbies 37

Chapter 3: Possible Effects Of Anxiety In Relationships And How To Stop Them 39

   Anxiety Can Break Down Connection And Trust .. 39
   Anxiety Can Crush Down Your True Voice And Create Panic 40
   Anxiety Can Make You Behave In a Selfish Way 41
   The Other Side Of Acceptance Is Anxiety 42
   Anxiety Can Rob Your Joy 43

How To Prevent Anxiety From Stealing The Magic Of Your Relationship? 44

   Recharging The Resources Of Emotion 45
   Allow Your Partner To Think Of You As A Support System 45
   Allow Your Partner To Take Part In Your Thoughts 46
   Ask For Reassurance 47
   Being Vulnerable 47
   Being Careful While Allowing Anxiety Into Your Relationship 48
   Analysis Can Result In Paralysis 49
   Pulling Closer And Pushing Away 50
   Having Tough Conversations Can Strengthen The Relationship 50
   Letting Your Partner The Things That Triggers You 51

Being Patient 51
Understanding The Need Of Your Partner's
Boundaries 52

Chapter 4: Strategies For Dealing With Relationship Anxiety 54

Where Does The Insecurity Originate From? 55
How Can Someone Deal With Relationship Anxiety? 56

Maintaining Self-Independence 57
Not Acting Out No Matter How Anxious
You Feel 58
Just Stop Measuring 59
Going All In 59

Simple Tips For Getting Rid Of Relationship Anxiety 60

Chapter 5: Self-Evaluation Of Relationship Anxiety 69

How To Find Out You Are Suffering From Anxiety
In Your Relationship? 70
Probable Causes Of Relationship Anxiety 73
How To Get Rid Of The Root Cause? 75
Self-Assessment Of A Relationship 77

Problem: Struggles Regarding Household
Responsibilities 79
Problem: Money 80
Problem: Not Keeping The Relationship On
The Priority List 82
Problem: Conflicts 83
Problem: Trust 85

Chapter 6: Identifying Various Behaviors That Can Trigger Anxiety 88

Definite Triggers Of Anxiety 92
How To Put An End To Such Behaviors? 93

An Effective Breathing Exercise 96
Step-By-Step Technique: Progressive Muscle
Relaxation.. 97
How To Put An End To Your Worries? 98
Ways Of Working Through Your Worries 100
- Getting Enough Sleep.. 101
- Writing It Down 101
- Following The Road Of Your Thoughts 102
- Picking Up Something That Can Be Controlled ... 103

Chapter 7: Relationship Conflicts 104
Primary Reasons For Relationship Conflicts 105
- Conflicts Rising From Professional Life 106
- Inappropriate Behavior And Infidelity 106
- When One Partner Fails To Meet The Expectation Of The Other.. 107

How To Deal With Relationship Conflicts? 108
- Examining Your Focus... 110
- Turning Conflicts Into Great Opportunities.......... 111
- Using Humor 112
- Practicing Acceptance.. 113
- Working On Forgiveness 114
- Communication 115
- Asking Right Questions... 116
- Making Time For Touch.. 117
- Try Being Direct 118
- Learn To Talk About Your Feelings Without Putting Blames On Your Partner 119
- Never Saying 'Never' or 'Always' 120
- Choosing Your Battles... 121

Not Objecting To The Complaints Of Your
Partner Automatically 121
Taking An Alternate Perspective 122
Not Showing Contempt 123
Not Getting Overwhelmed With Negativity 124
Knowing The Time For Time-Out 124

Chapter 8: Relationship Between Anxiety And Conflicts 126

Anxiety And Panic Attacks 127

Being Defensive 128
Shut Down 129

How To Successfully Overcome A Bad
Relationship Dispute? 129
Required Actions For Overcoming Conflicts
Between Partners 130
Compromising As A Common Solution 132

Agreeing To Disagree 133
When Is Compromise Regarded As An
Appropriate Move? 135
Resolving Disputes With The Help Of
Compromise 135

Chapter 9: Strategies For Improving Existing Relationships 137

Tips For Improving The Bond 144

Start By Asking Your Partner Something New 144
Fix A Month To Month Plan For Night Out 145
Expressing Appreciation 145
Changing The Timetable 146
Demonstrating Your Love 147

    Getting Familiar With The Behavior Of
    Your Partner 148
    Learning When To Say Sorry 149
    Going To Bed Together.. 150
    Being Honest All The Time 151
    Get Rid Of The Past 151

  Practical Exercises And Lessons 152

Chapter 10: Cultivating Healthy And Brand New Relationships... 169

  Allowing Vulnerability 169

  Selflessness 170

  Actual Beauty Comes From Inside............................ 171

  How To Cultivate A Meaningful Relationship In The Early Stages?.. 171

  Enjoying To Be In Love.. 177

  Useful Tips For A Happy And Long Relationship..... 178

  The Love Affair Errors.. 184

Chapter 11: Everyone Deserves A Wholesome And Healthy Relationship 187

  What Are The Aspects That Can Make A Relationship Healthy?... 189

    Developing The Links You Desire......................... 189

    Trusting Your Partner And Yourself...................... 190

Conclusion 191

Introduction

Congratulations on purchasing *Book Title,* and thank you for doing so.

Life is all about successful relationships. However, constant worry, along with anxious thoughts, can easily plague relationships. Anxiety is enough for tearing apart two people much before they can understand the wonder and essence of love. It might happen that you have lived your entire life within the boundaries of anxiety. Some recent events can also stir up all your underlying insecurities. But, there is no surety that your remaining life will be the same. All you need is to take back the lost control and kick anxiety out of your life. Everyone deserves a fulfilling and loving relationship in which there is no room for anxiety.

This book will help you and your partner tackle the prime issues of your relationship that can result in anxiety. There are various tools that you will need to build a lasting relationship. If you feel exhausted from living in a continuous state of anxiety, panic, and overwhelmed while being in a relationship, it is the right time to put an end to all your fears. Even if you are not in a relationship, but willing to establish a meaningful relationship in the future without any sign of anxiety, the exercises and practical life lessons in this book will provide you with all the confidence that you need.

There are plenty of books on this subject on the market, thanks again for choosing this one! Every effort was made to ensure it is full of as much useful information as possible, please enjoy!

Chapter 1: Understanding The Reasons Behind The Feelings Of Insecurity, Anxiety, And Attachment

While talking about relationships, there are various challenges that you will need to face and overcome. Anxiety is one such problem. It is an actual challenge, along with being a mental health disorder. If not checked on properly, it can lead to various problems that can harm your relationship. However, each and every one of us tend to develop feelings of anxiety at various times. It can be regarded as a serious issue in case it turns out to be severe. Anxiety can impact all your life relationships in a negative way. This can happen specifically if you tend to spend most of your time dealing with your worries and having thoughts about all those things that might go wrong or is already wrong in any relationship of yours. There are certain definite questions that might run across your mind when you tend to be excessively anxious in any relationship:

- What if the person is lying to me?
- Do they love me as much as I do?
- What if the person is cheating on me?
- Am I good enough for him/her?

- What would happen if we break up?
- Will he/she find someone more attractive than me?
- Can my anxiety destroy the relationship? (Anxiety about being anxious)

It is a normal thing to have all of these thoughts at some point of time in a relationship, specifically when the relationship is brand new. But, when such thoughts start to crop up in your mind very often, it might be a sign of an anxiety disorder or anxiety issues. The intensity of your rumination over the above-mentioned questions, along with some others that are quite similar, can determine the extent to which you have gone in your anxiety problem. It can also help in determining the extent of your insecurities in a relationship.

All of these thoughts of insecurity and anxiety get manifested in various physical ways. They are presented as symptoms such as insomnia, panic attacks, and shortness of breath. You will be able to find out that when you try to think in this way, a panic attack gets triggered in which the symptoms might be the fast beating of heart, shaking of your body, or a limp in the chest. These are some of the physiological signs that can indicate you have an anxiety disorder.

At times, all your anxiety thoughts might also encourage your relationship partner to start behaving in certain ways that can make you feel more stressed out. Such a thing can easily put a strain on your relationship. The main reason behind this is that you are excessively transparent in front of your partner that is allowing them to see your insecurities. This can easily provide them with an edge of manipulation over you. For example, they can change the perspective of certain events in a way that should not mean anything in normal to you but can start hurting you eventually.

You might start feeling anxious and worried about being the first to start a conversation most of the time. You might feel sick in your mind that your relationship partner might not like you as he/she never takes the initiative to start a conversation as much as you do. Such kind of anxiety tends to pile up and starts gathering the required momentum that can hurt the relationship.

Common Signs Of Relationship Anxiety

Love is a complicated topic for many people. But why? The reason behind this is that it can turn out to be the reason for our living as well as our reason for hopelessness. Relationship anxiety is something that keeps on checking the strength of love. Various signs can help you determine whether you are suffering from relationship anxiety or not. Let's have a look at them.

- **You keep on overanalyzing:** There is a thing: being critical or skeptical is not always bad. Actually, the capability of thinking thoroughly right before you start to believe in something can help you in discerning the reality from the picture of fiction. You can determine what the delusion is and what the fact is. Then, where is the issue? Well, the actual problem comes in the picture when you always feel dissatisfied with all the answers that you receive. You seem to feel incomplete even after cross-examining all the facts several times. A perfect example of this is when you start to set up scenarios in your mind and try to base all your actions on all those events that have not taken place yet.

Try to imagine this: you are on a lovely date. You give it your all for leaving a lasting impression on the other person. But, suddenly, you start asking the other person about their previous partners. You flood them with a pile of questions about their previous relationships. But do you know why you start doing this? All you are trying to do is to keep failure away. You are very afraid of failing. You want to gain knowledge about as many things as possible to make sure whether the other person will break your heart or not.

It is completely fine when you start expressing all your worries related to getting hurt in a relationship. What is not right is when you start disrespecting the other person by questioning them about very personal things. The worst part of all these is when you cannot block yourself from being analytical. That is what relationship anxiety is all about. You lose all your control over the negative thoughts related to your partner.

- **You feel scared to be in a sincere relationship:** According to you, how long should it take for two partners who are dating to be serious about their relationship? For some people, it might be after their third or fourth date. Some might even take weeks, months, or some years to be serious. The time required will generally depend on how well the two partners come to know each other. But, when you have relationship anxiety, your answer will most probably be "never". It does not matter whether you are in love with a person. Still, you won't be able to commit to that relationship. But why?

The reason behind this is your deep-seated fear, fear of being all alone in the end, fear of disappointment and betrayal. You might think that if you do not commit to someone, you will not get hurt. However, that is the illusion that is brought forward by your anxiety. As you try to stop yourself from committing to a relationship, you prevent yourself from learning the experiences. If you just focus on refusing the new chances to love, you will never come to learn about genuine love. Genuine love and relationship can help you to break through the barrier of relationship anxiety.

- **You are always attached to your partner:** Relationship anxiety will not only be providing you with a bad temper but will also be making you very needy. This is because you are paranoid. You are scared that even silence of two minutes between you and your partner can lead to your breakup. That is most unlikely to take place, but when it comes to relationship anxiety, your mind will always go in the opposite direction. So, how much attached can a person turn out to be who is suffering from relationship anxiety? The extent to which you can get attached to your partner will depend on your mind.

Here are certain examples that can indicate you are sensitive to certain cues that the other person will abandon you:

1. Replying to text messages as soon as possible and expecting the same.
2. Saying that you love your partner every ten minutes because you feel your partner might forget.
3. Feeling upset when the other person is going away for a business trip or something like that.
4. Looking for cuddles and hugs even when your partner is busy.

There is nothing wrong with asking for cuddles or saying that you love your partner. But, when you keep on doing the same repeatedly, it might turn out to be a bit annoying. This will ultimately make your love gestures look pointless and fake.

- **You always try to do something extra for pleasing your partner:** Genuine love is all about offering your attention and time to the other person. It is very romantic when you prepare a surprise lunch or dinner for your partner or just give them a visit at their workplace. However, when you are suffering from relationship anxiety, this might result to be a terrible thing.

You keep on doing something extra so that the other person does not lose their interest in you. You will try to do anything all the time to maintain your proper image. Even at times, when a single gesture can portray your love for your partner, you will think it is not at all enough. In place of maintaining a proper balance between love, career, and family, you put all your efforts into the relationship. You will slowly lose all your time for your family or yourself. You will lose your interest in your hobbies. When you just try to impress your partner, it might backfire massively. As you try to spoil the other person all the time, you will fail to improve yourself. This can make your partner feel that you are immature, and you are not at all ready for being in a committed relationship.

- **You lack self-confidence:** In various cases, people who suffer from relationship anxiety also suffer from a lack of confidence. It has been found that all those people who have low self-esteem tend to be more insecure in their relationships. To build up a relationship filled with joy and trust, both the partners are required to show that they are full of confidence in the partnership and arrangement.

For addressing your anxiety, you might think that it is better to go mute for some time. It might also force your relationship partner to start communicating with you, get in touch with you every now and then so that you can feel assured by knowing they care for you. It can also help you challenge all your irrational and anxious beliefs that your partner will not communicate first. However, this is not at all a healthy strategy. Fighting with the deep-rooted cause of your anxiety and gaining back your confidence is the only way to overcome your disorder. You will be able to lead a joyful and free life. Intimate relationships are, most of the time, emotionally intense. It is mostly because of the closeness that you tend to share with your partner. However, closeness of this type can also make you feel powerless and might lead your life to insecurity and anxiety.

Insecurity is the absence of confidence and self-doubt, while anxiety is the fear of something unknown. Majority of the times, insecurity gets aggravated into intense anxiety if not managed perfectly. You need to note that as you start worrying in a relationship, you will also develop low self-esteem. This is when insecurity settles in your life. You start to see the actions and intentions of your partner from a negative perspective.

Some of the most common symptoms related to intense anxiety disorder are:

- Tensed muscles
- Feeling restless
- Unable to remember or concentrate
- Unable to sleep properly
- Finding it difficult to make important decisions

Breeding Anxious Feelings And Thoughts

Relationships are always very pleasurable and beautiful. But they can breed in anxious feelings and thoughts. Such thoughts can crop up during any time in a relationship. Suppose you are single and thinking of getting into a serious relationship. In that case, the thought of getting in touch with the perfect person and starting a relationship can also ignite anxiety in you. You will need to learn how to control such feelings. Insecurity is nothing but a deep-seated feeling of feeling threatened or not being adequate in some ways. Every one of us feels it at some point in our lives. It is very normal to have certain feelings of self-doubt sometimes. However, insecurity of chronic type can hamper your life successes and put an end to your relationships.

When you suffer from excessive insecurity, you can feel peace going away from your life. You will not be able to get stay engaged with your relationship partner in an authentic and relaxed way. Some of the resultant actions that might arise from excessive insecurity include false accusations, jealousy, lack of trust, seeking for validation and reassurance, and snooping. Such attributes are not at all helpful for healthy relationships. They are powerful enough to push away your partner. They are many people who tend to believe that signs of insecurity are rooted in their relationship partners' actions. However, in reality, insecurity comes from your inside. You start arranging the blocks of insecurity inside yourself as you compare yourself negatively to other people. It can also initiate as you start harshly judging yourself with the inner voice.

Majority of the insecurities in relationships are completely based on fears and irrational thoughts that you are not that good like others. One thing that can be done from your side as you start noticing the uneasy feelings of insecurity is to take stock of all your values. Insecurity will always try to make you focus on all those things that you feel lacks in you. In most of the balanced relationships, both the partners bring in various qualities and strengths for complementing each other. For conquering your insecurities, try to take stock of all those values you offer in a relationship to your partner. A great character and personality are two such qualities that can maintain an overall relationship in a healthy way.

Building up your self-esteem also plays an important role in surmounting all the insecurities you face in a relationship. It is really important to feel good about yourself, about being the person you are to not seek for validation from another person. You complete yourself from the inside. You need to let your self-worth and independence shine bright through all your actions and deeds. When you become dependent on someone for your well-being, you hand over the key of your joy. You start to empower them. This whole thing might not be that healthy for a relationship. One of the best ways of building up your confidence is by silencing the inner critic and focusing all your attention and mind on the positive qualities. Try to look straight in the mirror and utter positive things to yourself. As you do this by looking in your own eyes, it can impact your mind and make you feel capable of love.

You also need to all your senses of self-identity and be capable of catering to all your personal needs. Suppose you were doing really well in catering to all your mental, physical, and emotional needs before being in a relationship. In that case, such things should not be stopped now as you have dedicated yourself to a relationship. You need to maintain your self-independence. You will need to stop yourself from turning into a person who is attached or needy.

Why Do You Feel Insecure, Attached, And Anxious In A Relationship?

As you start a new relationship, the starting phase can make you feel worried and also tensed up with various types of questions in your mind. You might start thinking: "Does my partner like me?", "Is this relationship going to work out?", or "How serious is my relationship going to get?" Unfortunately, such tensions and worries do not vanish in the later phases of a relationship when you are filled with anxiety. In actual, the more intimate and close you get to your partner, the more will be the intensity of your anxiety in such types of relationships.

Stress, anxiety, and worry related to your relationship can make you feel discouraged and lonely. You might also create a distance unknowingly between your partner and yourself. Another tragic consequence that might arise from anxiety is to dump all your beliefs about love. You might just give up all your hopes on love. So, it is very important to figure out why you feel anxious in your relationship and the reasons behind your attachment and insecurity.

As you fall in love, it can put demands on you in infinite ways, much more than you can really imagine. The more you start cherishing your partner, the more you will stand to lose them. The intense feeling that comes with love and powerful emotions can easily give birth to the fear of the unknown and the feeling of getting hurt in you. All these fears settle because of being treated in the way in a relationship as you wanted to be. As you start to feel and experience love in its actual way, or when you are being treated with excessive care and tenderness with which you are not familiar, anxiety sets in. Anxiety is not only the result of the events that take place between two partners in a relationship. It also depends on those things that you keep telling to your inner self and pour in your mind about all those events that slowly result in anxiety.

The biggest critic of your life is your inner mind, the 'mean coach' who is always trying to criticize you and flood you with all the bad advice that can easily trigger your fear of love and intimacy. It is your inner mind that keeps telling you:

- "You are not at all smart, and your partner will get bored with you."
- "You are not going to get someone who will love you, so stop trying."
- "Your partner does not love you at all. Get rid of the relationship before you are hurt."

Your mind is the responsible one that always tries to manipulate you. It can make you oppose yourself along with all those people whom you love. Hostility is encouraged by your mind, and you will soon find out that you are paranoid. You will start to eye and suspect all the moves of your partner. This will ultimately be reducing your self-esteem and will also be driving in the negative forces of jealousy, defensiveness, stress, anxiety, and distrust.

The main aim of the mean coach is to flood you with various types of thoughts that can easily eat up your happiness. You will end up worrying about the relationship instead of just enjoying the flow of the same. As you shift your focus from the relationship to the terrible thoughts, you will naturally get distracted from the actual relationship. You will be running away from love and proper communication with your love partner. You will soon find out that even the unnecessary issues are bothering you, and your mind is uttering destructive and nasty remarks. You might also develop a parental or childish attitude towards your partner. For instance, your relationship partner comes back home from work. He/she is not willing to have dinner as they are not feeling well. You are just sitting alone, and your inner critic gets activated. You will soon start thinking, "How can he/she refuse to have dinner with me?", "Was he/she out for dinner with someone else?", or "Can I really believe what he/she is saying?"

Such thoughts will keep breeding in your mind, and by the next morning, you are furious, temperamental, and insecure. You might get angry, and this, in turn, might make your partner defensive and frustrated. He/she will not even know what is running in your mind and will think your behavior is coming out of nowhere. So, it can be said that within a few hours, the dynamics of your healthy relationship have been shifted by you. In place of just enjoying all the time that you get with your partner, you might just waste a whole day with unnecessary thoughts. It will ultimately be building up a barrier between you two. The factor that is responsible for this sudden cyclone of events is not at all the situation itself. It has been done by the inner voice that was successful in clouding all your thoughts that ultimately took a disastrous path.

Your inner critical voice does not let you know that you are more resilient and stronger than you actually think of yourself. You can handle all the rejections, disappointments, and hurts that you are scared of. Human beings are built so that we can absorb all the negative situations, get healed from them, and deal with the same successfully. Our inner critical voice keeps on creating scenarios in our minds that do not even exist and will bring out all those threats that are not clear. The inner voice can easily misrepresent the actual reality of any situation.

The critical voice that we hear in our minds is the result of our own experiences and all those things to which we have successfully adapted to with time. As you start feeling insecure or anxious, you will tend to get overly attached and become desperate in all your actions. Control and possessiveness towards your relationship partner will set in. There are certain definite inner voices that speak up about you, your partner, and also the relationship. Such inner voices result from early attitudes to which you were exposed to amongst your family, friends, or in your society.

Critical Inner Voices About Relationship

- Majority of the people end up being hurt.
- Only a few relationships work out.

Critical Inner Voices About Your Partner

- You cannot trust your partner.
- He/she is most probably cheating on you.
- Most men are unreliable, selfish, and insensitive.

Critical Inner Voices Related To You

- You are the responsible one for everything that turns out to be bad.

- He/she is not interested in you.
- You will stay better on your own.

As you start listening to your inner voice, the final result is a relationship filled with anxiety that can easily destroy your live life in various ways. When you submit yourself to the anxiety, you will stop being the independent and strong person you used to be during the relationship's initial stages. This will ultimately be putting a serious strain on your relationship.

You might start feeling threatened by your anxiety, and you might end up controlling or dominating your partner. You will find yourself setting up rules for your partner for what they cannot do and what they can. This will be done on your part only to reduce the extent of your own insecurities. Sometimes, you might scream or yell at your partner without any kind of realization about the same.

Signs Related To Insecure Attachment

There are certain practices that result from insecure attachments. Let's have a look at them.

Very Demanding

You will not want your relationship partner to do something without you. You will try to stick to your partner. You will always request your partner for their consideration and time towards you, keeping aside all other relationships and friendships.

Jealousy Or Doubt

You will be very suspicious of the conduct of your partner. You will be questioning their connections and also to whom your partner communicates with. You will feel jealous of any person who gets close to your partner.

Enthusiastic Dependency

You will depend on your partner for the prosperity of your enthusiasm. You will find that your joy comes up from the relationship.

Anger Issues

You might get angry with your partner without any reason. If not addressed in the proper way, this can adversely affect the relationship.

You can fight your insecurities by uncovering the roots and finding the actual reason behind your actions. Try to challenge your inner voice and just let your relationship flow freely.

Chapter 2: Reasons Behind Irrational Behaviors Resulting From Anxiety

Love is initiated with a huge bursting of hormones in our brain that tends to interrupt our normal behaviors. Love has the power of making us feel crazy, drive us wild, and distract us. When you start being irrational, you will not be able to listen to logic, reason, or even apply your common sense. All you want is to meet a particular need of yours, no matter in which way it can be achieved. Until you meet that need of yours, you will keep acting in an unpredictable and terrific way. You need to remember that our emotions form a very important aspect of all our lives. It can not only influence wellness, but it can also determine the relationships with various people. At times, you might feel overwhelmed because of all your negative emotions, no matter how hard you try to keep them under check. Emotions take into play the complex states of our minds that can affect our bodies, along with the external environment.

The emotions that you feel are the perception of all those events that are taking place around you. All these emotions force you to portray several behavioral patterns. When you feel upset with someone or something, you might lash out and become angry. When you feel unhappy and overwhelmed, you start crying. Similarly, when you experience positive love emotions, you might show affection. When something seems funny, you start laughing. Your capability to understand and control all your emotions and its responses is a very important skill that can affect relationships with other people. If you just concentrate on expressing the negative emotions, your health and relationships will be at risk. Irrational behavior can be described as an array of intense emotions in certain situations where your partner cannot understand the need for such strong emotion.

In romantic relationships, our emotions run wild, along with misunderstandings that are often triggered by such emotions. The main reason behind this attached relationship. When approached in the perfect way, attached relationship can foster love, comfort, and security. However, if both the partners are not responsive to one another's needs, such a relationship might turn out to be unstable. Whenever you feel that your relationship security is being threatened, you might respond with very strong emotions like loneliness, grief, disappointment, and anger. When all these responses are expressed intensely, they might seem irrational. Science cannot tell you the exact definition of love, but it can tell you what love can do. When you are in love, the processes of molecular, sensory, and organic chemistry, along with sexual union, can make people do certain foolish and crazy things.

Romantic feelings, attraction, and aroused love that are most often experienced during the initial stages of a relationship are also characterized by targeted attention, obsessive behavior, and intense desire. It is the stage of affection when people seem to act the most impulsive, irrational, and emotional. It shows somewhat similar effects like the mind frame of addiction. The intense feeling of a genuine bond with someone, the sense of peace, calm, and stability caused by this bond, is associated to the hormones that get discharged with the birth of a child, production of milk, and orgasm. So, no matter how sensible is the chemistry of a couple, it will still be having some dangerous emotional and behavioral results. Love is very natural for human life, just like breathing. When you try to prevent the same out of discomfort or fear, it might turn out to be suffocating.

Irrational Behaviors Resulting From Anxiety

Anxiety can successfully alter the chemistry of your brain. It can trigger emotions and behaviors that would never occur to you under normal conditions. But when anxiety takes control, everything seems to go out of control. Let's have a look at some behaviors that can crop up when a stressful trigger or tough situation comes in a relationship.

Unwarranted Irritability

We human beings get irritated. It is quite natural. You might be hungry or have had a bad day at work, or some other reason. Irritability cannot be termed as irrational until and unless it comes from anxiety. The response of fight or flight that boosts up all the hormones can make us stand at the edge. It can lead to irritation from no definite cause except for anxiety. One of the unfortunate aspects of irritability is that it can be easily directed at our loved ones. Whenever irritability of irrational kind crops up and forces you to burst open at your partner, it might be very difficult for you to explain your reason for doing so. You might not have any idea where this mood of yours is originating from. It can lead you to conclude that you must be mad at the other person for any reason. Now it seemed like a perfect time for expressing all your anger.

Your partner will have no idea about what wrong they did. Right before you come to know the actual reason, it will form a barrier between you two. The reason for your initial anxiety will not be of any concern now as the irritation resulting from the same made all the damage.

Compulsive Behavior

Anxiety can often be found at the base of compulsive behavior that also includes obsession. You want to have in control some aspects of your environment. So, you try to develop certain habits and routines that can offer you with an outward appearance of the order. The relationship uncertainties can often lead to several anxious thoughts regarding the future. So, you just engage yourself in compulsive behaviors that can provide you with a little bit of power for controlling a small part of your own life and the future. Such behaviors can be anything out of which some common ones are checking the door lock number of times, need to keep everything in a particular order, making sure the gas burner is off several times before you leave the house, and many others.

Excessive Worrying

Every one of us worries. It is very natural. Our lives are completely unpredictable. This is the main reason why anxiety seems to be so prevalent. But when that specific worry starts overtaking your mind's thoughts to an extent when you cannot even think of something else, it is a problem. After checking out some weird text, you might feel certain worry much before you can start thinking regarding the situation in a rational way. He/she loves me a lot, I trust them completely, and I am sure I will not get hurt by them. There is no need to jump right to any obvious conclusion. In case you are dealing with anxiety, this whole situation will trigger more than just a simple moment of worry.

You will feel your mind getting filled with several small and large pieces of messages from the past, whether innocent or not. You will try to scan your partner's actions in your mind to identify the moments when you felt suspicious. Your worry gets turned into a state of panic that ultimately leads you to the kingdom of irrational thoughts. However, if this situation is happening for the first time, and you cannot recall anything from the past, that is exactly when your behaviors will seem irrational. Regardless of the outcome, thinking and worrying to the boundary of panic aren't going to provide you with all the answers that you need. To stop worrying, you will need to release all those things that you cannot control.

Physical Aggression

When the response of fight or flight gets triggered, some of the reactions might turn out to be violent. As you feel that you are in danger or threatened, your body will take over the control for protecting you. When you face a situation that triggers your anxiety, in case the severity is excessive, there are chances that you will express your anxiety in physical ways. For emotionally protecting yourself, you try to arm yourself physically. You might not find any sense in the behavior, even though you are displaying that behavior. That is all that makes the behavior look irrational.

Moping

This might look less drastic when compared to aggression or irritability. But it might turn out to be detrimental. Moping is generally characterized by depression, sadness, and also lack of energy. This is the result of anxiety that shuts down your body and mind. Your mind will feel tired, just like your limbs. Depression of this sort results in sadness that seems like emerging from nowhere. The only thought you might have in your mind is, "I don't feel the urge to do it." This 'it' can be anything. This form of depressive mood is enough for straining a healthy relationship, specifically when your partner does not have any clear idea if they have done something wrong.

Need For Understanding Your Partner

Every one of us desires to be seen, understood, and heard. All of us want this, especially from our relationship partners. We desire our partners to say, "I am listening to you", "I can understand your pain", or "Yes, I can get it what you are trying to say." The capability of understanding the emotional well-being of your partner is very important for developing a healthy relationship. When you can identify your partner's emotions or the reason behind their behaviors, you will be able to respond to the needs of your partner effectively. This will allow you to offer your partner with the perfect support. You will be able to say the perfect things in perfect situations.

One cannot overemphasize the importance of understanding the partner's opinions, views, and perspectives, specifically at the time of disagreements. The best way of developing a proper understanding of your partner's emotions is by asking them regularly how they feel, the reason behind their feeling, and what their feeling can be compared with. It can help you when you are unsure of your partner's emotions or reasons behind their behaviors. For doing a great job at understanding the emotions of your partner, you will need to understand your feelings as well. You will need to be stable emotionally. As you improve your emotional self-awareness, you can also motivate your partner to do the same.

While talking about emotions, you will need to understand that it might not be very easy for your companion or partner to express all their feelings to you. The confidence and trust level that your partner has over you will determine how much feelings they can actually share with you. It is very important to establish a general network of trust in a healthy relationship. No one can deny that effective communication is the only key to a successful relationship. So, it is very important to communicate all your thoughts and feelings as much as possible with your partner. This can help in enhancing the level of confidence and trust in your relationship. Understanding is always regarded as one of the greatest qualities of a perfect partner in any successful relationship. We all want someone who can understand us completely.

Also, you need to be careful while imposing all your beliefs and ideals on your relationship partner. No matter how better you think of yourself than your partner when it comes to maturity, intellect, or even experience. Do not try to force your world views on the other person. You need to learn to respect the other person's point of view, their situations, and perspectives in general. One of the surest ways of understanding your partner and making your relationship work in the best possible way is acknowledging and understanding that your relationship is not at all the only thing in this universe. The same thing applies to your partner as well.

You will need to maintain and improve the kind of life you had before starting the relationship. There is no need to force your partner to place your relationship on the priority list. You need to provide your partner with all the freedom they need to have fun, to live, and be happy in their way. It does not matter if you are always around them or not. Do not stop your partner for going out with their friends, let them socialize, allow them to travel wherever they feel like solo, and let them live their own lives on their own terms. Do not just push yourself upon your partner all the time. Try to encourage your partner to opt for their personal goals and pursue self-development. This will make your partner gain more confidence in your relationship. In turn, this will ultimately increase the level of affection that your partner has for you.

For effective understanding, you will first need to learn to compromise. You will need to feel encouraged to find out a common ground, which is a basic aspect of compromising. There is no need to point out that you are right all the time. One thing that you will need to remember, both of you are sailing in the same boat with a common goal. Both of you are not enemies but progressive partners. Another effective and beautiful way of understanding your partner is by providing them with the chance to explain their situations and themselves. Do not just react suddenly before they can explain what is wrong or what happened. You will need to guard your emotions and heart in a diligent way. Whenever you feel that your partner disappointed you or made you upset, just give them an opportunity to explain their situation.

Yes, it might indeed sound a bit challenging to understand your partner, especially in situations when you feel they are wrong. It always hurts the most when you feel let down and betrayed. No matter what the case is, you will have to regain the love and strength to listen. You will need to be a sincere listener. Also, trust plays a very important role in this aspect so that your partner can take you through their road of motivation and intention for all their acts. A relationship is bound to thrive when both the partners tolerate and understand each other.

Instead of just getting upset in certain situations, you can opt for showing some maturity. In case you feel offended by the actions of your partner, do not just start a fight. Try to explain your point of view and why you feel they offended you. Try to let your partner know that you have forgiven them, but you are just willing to let them know. Being annoyed will do nothing other than worsening the whole situation.

Lack Of Understanding – The Prime Reason Behind Relationship Failures

Understanding in a relationship matters a lot. It is the main reason why the majority of the relationships tend to fail after a certain point of time. Just when you start a new relationship, whether dating or newly married, the first thing that both partners need to do is to examine each other's behavior. Try to ask questions in case you have any doubt. When you ask your partner direct questions, they will feel the urge to open up their feelings to you. In case your partner offends you, try not to keep any grudges. The capability to forgive and settle things cheerfully every time you get offended by your partner is one of the supporting pillars of relationships.

You can try to encourage your partner to open up about their feelings and behaviors to you, regardless of the situation. Human beings might sometimes find it a bit difficult to relay their feelings and idea into words. This might turn out to be a challenge in romantic relationships. In such situations, being patient is the best possible solution. You can try to give them the motivation to open up and discuss various issues that concern your relationship. Doing this will assure your partner that you are willing to listen to them. This will ultimately help you to in flourish your relationship. Understanding the feelings and emotions of people is not at all simple, especially in romantic relationships. You have to continuously make an effort to be in tune with your partner's state of mind and emotions.

Sometimes, it might happen that the other person is feeling upset for some reason, which they themselves cannot understand. But still, they will expect that you will understand their concern. You might say that you cannot read minds. However, all you can do is stay calm and assure your partner that you understand what is bothering them. A very effective way of removing all kinds of tensions is by unleashing all the worries at one time to your loved one. This might turn out to be very overwhelming but is counterproductive as well. You will need to understand that emotional connection is a street with two ways. You will need to put in all your efforts to understand your partner's emotions to reciprocate their effort to understand your emotions.

Control Your Body Language And Manners

In case both the partners try to raise their voice at the time of an argument, relaxing the situation and understanding each other will turn out to be challenging. You need to pay all your attention to the tone and volume of your voice. When the pitch of your voice goes above the normal level, you will find it difficult to listen to or understand your partner. Mannerisms and body language also play an important role. The body language that you possess at the time of an argument will directly affect the way in which your partner responds. You will make it tough for your partner to understand all your needs. For example, if you stand crossing your arms, you will portray yourself as being defensive. Your body needs to reflect the desire to communicate from your side.

Make Communication A Daily Habit

For better communication, you can try to cultivate a daily habit of relaying your feelings regarding any situation along with your relationship in general. There is no need to keep waiting until and unless there is an issue in your relationship. Both partners will need to establish an environment where it is completely fine to speak up about their feelings. A great way of doing so is by asking questions of open-ended nature. For example, "How was your day, and what was the best moment?" In this way, you can encourage your partner to speak up more about themselves. You will also be able to establish meaningful conversations without any extra effort.

Not Forcing Your Partner To Change

Let your partners be the way they are. Do not pressurize them to change. When you try to change your partner or alter their feelings, you will be harming the relationship. When you speak up about your own feelings, try to portray your partner as a medium of sharing your feelings and emotions. Make it clear that all you want is to be heard and understood. Do not apportion blame, and do not rely on pressure. You will need to let your partner know that you are not telling them to fix anything. If your partner tries to fix any critical situation, it can mount excessive pressure on them. Just try to make yourself clear in front of them.

Choosing The Perfect Time

You are required to choose a perfect time when you want to communicate with your partner about your emotions. Considering your partner's mood and their state of mind right before you initiate an emotional conversation is very important. Do not try to communicate when your partner is piled up with work, feeling sleepy, or spending time with their friends. One thing that you will need to keep in mind is that everyone does not communicate in the same way. Try to figure out how your partner communicates and make them understand your way of communication as well. Another important thing that you will need to keep in mind while communicating is to be stable. Do not communicate when you are excessively emotional.

Practical Ways Of Getting To Know Your Partner In A Better Way

There are certain ways in which you can learn about your partner very easily. Here are some of them.

Spending Time With Their Friends

Spending time with friends of your partner is a great way of understanding them. As you hang out with your partner's friends, you might see a different side of them.

If your relationship is new, hanging out with your partner's friends is the perfect way of learning about your partner. Whenever your partner asks you to go out with their friends, just say yes.

Plan A Vacation

If you are willing to understand the true self of your partner, try to plan and go for a vacation together. It does not matter even it is for a weekend only. You will get to spend some time alone with your partner and will also get the chance to communicate with them. Also, you will come to know the way they react to complexities. For instance, the way in which he/she reacts to a flight delay. As you experience new things together, you will be able to take your relationship to a whole new level. You can come to know about the interests of your partner. In simple terms, you can get a look at the true raw image of your partner.

Sharing Hobbies

You know that your partner loves reading books. However, do you have any idea of what he/she is reading? Try to show interest in the hobbies of your partner. This way, you can also encourage your partner to show interest in your hobbies. Relationships can be regarded as a very intimate friendship in which commonalities play a vital role. You might not find reading books interesting, but try to have some knowledge about the passions and hobbies of your partner.

Chapter 3: Possible Effects Of Anxiety In Relationships And How To Stop Them

Anxiety can take a toll on your health – physical, mental, and emotional. But, have you ever considered the effects of anxiety in your relationship? Anxiety can lead to overwhelming feelings, fear, a sense of tension and unease, and periods of panic. It comes with the capability of taking over all your thoughts and just bleeds into all parts of your normal life. In case you feel that your relationship is being strained due to some reason, anxiety might turn out to be one of the root causes. Can your partner's anxiety or yours push your relationship towards extreme risk? Here's how anxiety strains relationships.

Anxiety Can Break Down Connection And Trust

Anxiety often leads to worry or fear that might reduce your awareness of all the true needs in any given situation or moment. Not only that, but anxiety can also make you less aware of your partner's needs and wants. In case you feel worried about what exactly is happening, you will find it much more difficult to figure out what is happening. As you feel overwhelmed, there are chances that your partner might not feel your presence in difficult situations.

So, what can be done in this regard? You will need to train your mind to start living in the moment. In case you figure out a concern or fear that is making all your thoughts to create a distance from the current situation or facts, just pause and think. Try thinking all those things that you already know in opposition to what is not known to you. Calm yourself down right before you start to act. You can start taking purposeful steps in order to build back the lost trust in your partner. Try to share with your partner openly every time as you feel tensed or worried. Reach out to your partner consciously, either verbally or physically, when in the normal case, you might just attack or draw yourself back in fear.

Anxiety Can Crush Down Your True Voice And Create Panic

People who suffer from anxiety might feel troubled while expressing their true feelings. It might also be very difficult for them to set up reasonable boundaries by directly asking for the space or attention that they need. As anxiety experiences are not at all comfortable, you might try to delay the experiences of the same subconsciously. On the contrary, anxiety can also make you believe that you need to talk about something right away, whereas it would be beneficial if a short break is taken. When you do not want to express what you need or feel, the effects of anxiety on your relationship tends to be stronger.

You will find out your emotions spiraling out of control eventually as you keep them buried inside yourself. You might become defensive as well as overwhelmed. What can be done to take care of such problems? Try acknowledging all that you feel as soon as possible instead of just keeping them away for later. A concern or feeling is not required to be a big disaster for addressing the same. Try to approach your partner with all your concerns in a kind way. Make sure you are not panicking or procrastinating. Take out some time for your own good to easily unpack some of the major fears or thoughts that are going on in your mind. When not addressed at the right time, it can easily drain all your energy and time in the relationship.

Anxiety Can Make You Behave In a Selfish Way

As anxiety is nothing but an overactive response to fear, a person who is experiencing it might focus, most of the time, on their problems or concerns. All your fears and worries can easily put extra pressure on your healthy relationship, which can be regarded as unnecessary. You might develop the feeling that you are required to worry all the time to protect yourself in the relationship. However, the actions and thoughts of this kind might keep you at a distance from being vulnerable and compassionate with your partner.

In case your partner gets anxious as well, you might start building up resentment and just react selfishly. The perspectives and attitudes that you will develop might turn out to be contagious. You find it difficult to keep your stress level under proper control, especially in situations when your partner is defensive, feeling upset, or anxious. Try to attend properly to all your needs. Do not just give all your attention to the fears. Whenever you find yourself getting defensive or fearful, just take some moment to consider the amount of compassion you have for your partner and yourself. Directly ask for all the support that you are looking for to feel understood and loved. Just apologize to yourself for allowing anxiety to make yourself self-absorbed.

The Other Side Of Acceptance Is Anxiety

As you worry, you will get a signal that will tell you something is not right. You might feel the signal from your brain's sudden tight feeling or a sudden pull at your chest. The signal that you get helps you in acting in the perfect way. For example, when you stand up for a person who is being poorly treated. Unhealthy anxiety levels will make you feel that you are carrying an emotional rock all the time in your stomach. It will make you reject all those things that are not at all dangerous. You will keep on avoiding those things that can benefit you. Anxiety can also prevent you from taking some healthy actions in order to change certain things in your love life that is hurting you.

Just try practicing being uncomfortable. There is no need to obsess over or ignore any of your uncomfortable thoughts. Try to take as many constructive actions as possible. Sometimes all that your partner wants from you is to be present for his or her feelings. You might need to offer yourself the same gift at times. Take the initiative to show your partner that you are present for them. It can be done with a soft touch or soft eyes. At the same time, try to be present for yourself as well with a soft breath.

Anxiety Can Rob Your Joy

To experience joy in its true form, you will need a sense of freedom or safety. Anxiety will make you feel either limited or fearful. Also, a body and brain trained to extreme stress will face a tough time enjoying some private time and intimacy. Fears and negative thoughts can easily impact a person's ability to be in the moment within a healthy relationship. It will be sucking out all the joy from the moments potentially.

Try not to take yourself very seriously. Using your sense of humor can help in overcoming anxiety very well. Remember to play and spend some time with your companion. Laugh together with your partner. Joy comes with the power of physically comforting and healing the brain in various ways that are essential for a relationship's health.

How To Prevent Anxiety From Stealing The Magic Of Your Relationship?

Intimate relationships are, more or less, like clear mirrors. They help us in reflecting the worst side and the best side of us. They come with the power of inflaming all our struggles or can soothe them. When everything seems to be right, it will seem like smooth magic. Even when everything looks to be perfect in a relationship, anxiety can crop up and steal all the magic. It will lead to the loosening of a perfect connection between two partners who are meant to be together. Relationships of all kinds need tenderness, trust, vulnerability, and patience. People who suffer from anxiety often come with all these qualities for providing to a relationship. However, anxiety can also erode all of them very quickly.

In case you are struggling with relationship anxiety, there are various things related to you that can make loving you a lot easier. Every relationship struggles at some point of time. When anxiety comes into play, the struggle might take a different turn. Anxiety can function in various ways and will affect different relationships in different ways. Here are some definite ways that can help you to strengthen the bond of your relationship and also provide it with all the protection against anxiety.

Recharging The Resources Of Emotion

If you are suffering from anxiety, you are probably very sensitive to the requirements of other people. You try to dedicate everything to the relationship. However, sometimes anxiety can exhaust all those resources from your relationship at the same pace as you invest them. It is quite natural. There various things that will come with all those resources so that you can mend up all the gaps. But you will also need to recharge all those resources whenever you can. Try to provide your partner with all your attention, affection, gratitude, touch, and conversation whenever you are around your partner. It can help in reducing the effect of anxiety in your relationship.

Allow Your Partner To Think Of You As A Support System

Your partner will hesitate most of the time to pile up all their worries on you. It might be the case, especially when your partner's worries are not as big as yours. People who suffer from relationship anxiety come with lots of strength. So, make sure your partner knows that you are present for them all the time. No matter how small or big is their struggle; you can always be the support system for your partner. A relationship is all about providing support to each other in all situations. However, that does not mean you will neglect all your worries. Try to handle your struggles and your partner's as well at the same time. Try to be deliberate to turn yourself into a rock at times. Ask for it, hold, and touch. Nothing can be more healing than the warmth of your partner's love.

Allow Your Partner To Take Part In Your Thoughts

Anxious thoughts are indeed very personal. However, try to allow your partner to share some space in your thoughts. It is an essential part of an intimate relationship. You might keep on thinking about what can be done on your side for feeling safe, what could go wrong, and what is bad for you. You might also keep thinking about other people. But always make sure that you allow your partner in all those thoughts that arrests you. When you try to keep all your things excessively to yourself, it will very easily widen the distance between you and your partner. There is nothing wrong with sharing the things that worry you with your partner.

You might come up with a brand new way of dealing with your worries as you share them with your partner.

Ask For Reassurance

Anxiety has the habit of cropping up in every situation of life. When you forget to check on your anxiety, it can indulge you in doubting all those things that do not even need to be doubted, for example, your relationship. It is absolutely okay and quite normal to ask for reassurance from your partner. But make sure you keep the same under control. Asking for it too much might portray you as a needy person. Neediness is often regarded as the greatest enemy of desire. With time it can suppress the spark. Make sure that you provide your partner with the opportunity of loving you without any conditions. Do not prompt now and then to get loved. Allowing things with the flow will make the experience lovely for your partner and also better for you.

Being Vulnerable

Anxiety can affect your relationship in various ways. For some people, it might also stir the need for continuous reassurance. For others, it can make them feel like holding back. Vulnerability is the act of being transparent to one another. It is quite beautiful and can provide you with the essence of a healthy and successful relationship. When you try to protect yourself excessively, you might just invite the rejection that you are seeking protection for. The basic aspect of intimacy is to allow your partner to get close to you compared to the rest of the world. It is all about trusting your partner in showcasing the messy, untamed, and fragile parts of you. A person who loves you truly will always accept the messy side of yours, the parts that are sometimes baffling, and sometimes beautiful.

You might feel scared in opening up all those parts of yours to others. However, when you showcase them in front of someone who loves you, the worries will look like worries only, not realities. You will feel loved, and with time, you will be okay.

Being Careful While Allowing Anxiety Into Your Relationship

There is nothing specific that can trigger your anxiety. That is the most awful thing about anxiety. It will search for a target, a strong anchor, so that it can hold itself in place. If you are in a healthy and intimate relationship, that is the point where anxiety will try to anchor itself. Intimate relationships can very easily draw anxiety into it using its gravitational pull. It will ultimately give birth to the feelings of jealousy, doubt, insecurity, and suspicion. Anxiety can turn out to be a villain in this way. You are making your relationship an easy target by yourself. Try to remind yourself that because you are feeling worried, there is nothing that you will need to worry about. Worry only when you think you need to. Try seeing it the way it is, anxiety, and nothing truth. Your partner loves you. Just let that be the only truth. That will be enough for holding you.

Analysis Can Result In Paralysis

There is a very famous saying – 'Analysis Can Result In Paralysis.' Yes, it is true. Is it lust or love? Am I making a fool out of myself? How will it work if we both do not like the same food/ music/ books/etc.? What if my partner breaks my heart and goes away? What if my partner gets sick of me? What if our holiday flight gets canceled? All these are very common analysis that can be seen in our daily lives, especially when you suffer from anxiety. The things on which you put all your focus are the things that will gain importance in your life. So, when you try to focus on the problems, they will be absorbing all your energy until they get powerful enough to create something big. They will be draining your capability to sense fun and love. What can be done is dealing with this? Here is something that will work. Try to set a particular time frame when you can act like everything will be in order and will be fine. For example, you can worry from 08:00 A.M. till 02:0 P.M. every day. After that time frame is over, try to let go of all your worries and start acting as everything is fine.

You are not required to believe what you are assuming. Just act in the opposite direction. You will get a new chance to worry the next day again if you require to. Try to guide yourself with the evidence, and not with the worries that haunt you every night.

Pulling Closer And Pushing Away

When you try to focus on everything, the chances are high that things will get wobbly. You will start focusing on all those things that are not perfect in relation to your partner or the relationship. At the same time, you will look for reassurance that your partner is committed and loves you. It will make you push away your partner. Right after that, you will pull your partner close to you again for reassurance. Try to discuss the same with your partner. If this process seems familiar, try to figure out when it is happening along with your partner. When such things happen, do not take them as criticism. It is your partner who is asking for stability in the relationship and how you both love each other.

Having Tough Conversations Can Strengthen The Relationship

Every relationship needs to deal with tough things now and then. However, anxiety can make everything look more threatening than they are. You might think of not talking to your partner about complex issues. The reason behind this is your fear, 'What will happen to the relationship after this conversation?' Difficult things are not bound to go away. They stick to their place until they start boiling. Try to have trust in yourself and your partner. Both of you can easily cope up with any kind of tough decision. The secret is both of you will need to give in the same effort. Trust builds the base of relationships. Trusting your relationship that it can fight through tough conversations is very important.

Letting Your Partner The Things That Triggers You

Is there are specific situation or action when your anxiety gets triggered? Strangers? Being Late? Crowds? Loud Music? No matter what it is, try to discuss about the same with your partner. Talking about anxiety triggers can help your partner understand whenever you are in any problem. He/she will be able to understand what exactly is happening to you whenever you face any of the triggers. It will also help you to get all the reassurance that you need at the time of worry. You will be able to make your relationship stronger than before.

Being Patient

For feeling better or for easing out your anxiety, you might feel tempted to opt for a quick fix to an issue or a problem in your relationship. You might find yourself getting frustrated with your partner's desire to just wait or just keep on talking about the problem. However, you need to understand that your romantic partner may also see things differently, much clearer than you. Relax yourself, take time, and be patient. Opting for a simple quick fix is not the solution. Just try to be in the conversation with your partner patiently. It will ultimately be helping your relationship.

<u>Understanding The Need Of Your Partner's Boundaries</u>

To keep the relationship healthy, connected, and happy, boundaries that are built by your partner can help a lot. You will need to understand that the boundary lines drawn by your partner are not their way of keeping you out. It is a form of self-protection so that they do catch your anxiety. As you suffer from anxiety, you might feel worried about something and want to discuss the same with your partner over and over again. However, that isn't going to do any good for you or your relationship. Your partner loves you. They can draw a bold line between the very last time when you discussed something and the next time when you are going to. Talking is indeed a healthy way of communication. But when you keep repeating the same thing now and then, it might turn out to be draining. It can give birth to a serious issue just because you keep talking about an issue that isn't there.

The boundaries drawn by your partner is important for nurturing love and also for making it grow. Try talking to your partner regarding what they need for feeling okay in the context of your anxiety. Do not just try to break through the boundaries. Instead of doing pushing against the boundary line, try to invite them. It can help in keeping the connection loving and strong. It will also provide your partner with a feeling that they can still preserve a sense of themselves without being piled up by the worries from your side.

Chapter 4: Strategies For Dealing With Relationship Anxiety

Every one of us has seen ourselves at one or either side of the scenario: either the worrier or the worrier's partner. There are chances that some people have even experienced both. Anxiety and insecurity can turn out to be toxic to the closest and dearest relationships. Although it can bounce back and forth from one partner to another, the root of our insecurity and its cure can be found deep inside us.

According to some studies, people who have low self-esteem tend to suffer more from relationship insecurity. It can prevent them from fully experiencing the positive sides of a strong and loving connection. People who come with low self-esteem will not only want to see their partner in a better light than themselves, but in the moments when they doubt themselves, they find it tough to even recognize the affirmations of their partner. When the insecurities are acted out, it can push your partner away from you. And thus resulting in a self-fulfilling prophecy. As this struggle is internal and keeps going on the majority of the time, it is essential to deal with the worries and insecurities without dragging or distorting your partner into them. All of these can be achieved by taking two simple steps:

- Find out the root cause of the insecurity
- Throw a challenge to the inner critic that tries to sabotage the relationship

Where Does The Insecurity Originate From?

Nothing in this world can awaken distant hurts like a serious relationship. Relationships can easily stir up all our old feelings from the past in comparison to anything else. Even our brains get flooded with similar neurochemicals in both situations. Every one of us possesses working models for our relationships that get formed automatically from all our early days of attachment to influential caretakers. The early patterns can easily give our adult relationships the required shape. The style of attachment that we possess helps influence which partner we select to be with and the dynamics that are going to play in the relationship. An attachment pattern that is secure enough can help one to be more self-possessed and confident. However, when a person comes with a preoccupied or anxious attachment style, there are chances that they will feel insecure in the relationship and also towards their partner.

It is important to know our style of attachment. It can help in realizing various ways that we might recreate any dynamic from the past. Realizing our attachment style can help in forming a better relationship and also choose better partners. It will ultimately alter the style of attachment that we possess. Lastly, it can provide us with an idea about how insecure feelings might be misplaced, based on past events compared to the current situation.

Relationships are strong enough to shake us up. They tend to challenge all our core feelings that we have regarding ourselves. They can take us out of the comfort zones. They might also increase our inner critic's volume and reopen all the wounds that are unresolved from the past. It can be said that what we felt and experienced in our past days can easily affect our current relationships. If we can successfully alter the attachment pattern, we can start a healthy relationship with the correct partner.

How Can Someone Deal With Relationship Anxiety?

For challenging all our insecurities and worries, we will need to have proper knowledge about our inner voice. You will need to try your level best to catch it every time it tries to creep into your mind. Sometimes, it might turn out to be a lot easy. Suppose you are getting decked up for going on a date with your partner. Suddenly, your inner voice crops up, "You are so fat. You are looking disgusting! Try to cover yourself; otherwise, he/she will not get attracted to you." It might sometimes turn out to be sneaky, while sounding soothing, "Just be you. There is no need to show him/her how you feel. You will not get hurt." This inner voice of yours can even portray your partner in such a way that will be making you feel even more insecure – "He/she is not a person whom you can trust. He/she is going to cheat on you."

Identifying your critical voice is the initial step of challenging it. When you start challenging your inner critical voice, you must also try to take various actions that work against all the voice's directives. While talking about a relationship that indicates not to act out relying on the unwarranted insecurities or just acting out in ways that we do not even respect. Let's have a look at some of the helpful steps that can be taken by you.

Maintaining Self-Independence

When in a relationship, it might seem a bit tough to keep a small sense of our own selves separated from that of our partners. A healthy relationship aims to prepare a tasty fruit salad and not a blended smoothie. In simple terms, you should not forget about the essential parts that you possess for getting merged as a couple. You must work on yourself to maintain all the unique aspects that made your partner feel attracted to you. All of this needs to be maintained even when the relationship ages. In this simple way, you will be able to hold strong, with the knowledge that you are still a whole person in and of yourself.

Not Acting Out No Matter How Anxious You Feel

You might feel that this is much easier to say that being done. However, we all know that the insecurities we possess can easily lead to destructive behavior. Act of possessiveness or jealousy can hurt your partner. Checking their text messages, getting mad whenever they look at someone else, call now and then for checking on them – all such acts can be avoided from your side no matter how anxious you feel. If you can do this successfully, you will feel more trusting and stronger in your relationship. More importantly, you will turn out to be more trustworthy.

As you can only alter half of the dynamic, it is always helpful to keep thinking about all those actions taken by you that can push away your partner. If you act in a definite way that you respect and still do not feel like getting all you want, it is better to make a conscious decision to discuss the same with your partner. You can also try to change the situation. But there is no need to feel victimized or just let yourself act in certain ways that you do not respect.

Just Stop Measuring

There is no need to assess or constantly evaluate the moves of your partner. You need to accept the fact that your partner is a completely different person compared to you with an autonomous mind. You won't be seeing things or just express your love for your partner in the same way. However, this does not mean at all that you should settle for someone in a relationship who cannot offer you all that you want from a healthy relationship. A successful relationship is required to be equal in terms of kindness and maturity that is exchanged. In case things seem to be off, you can communicate about the same to your partner. You can clearly say what you want from them. But it won't be right if you want your partner to read your mind and find out what you want. As soon as you start the blame game, it takes the form of a vicious cycle, which is hard to break free.

Going All In

Every human being has anxiety. However, you can try to improve your overall tolerance for the various kinds of ambiguities presented inevitably by your relationship simply by being absolutely true to your own self. We tend to invest in all those people even after knowing that they can hurt us. As you keep one foot out of the door, it can keep the relationship from getting excessively intimate and might undermine it. As you take a chance without allowing the insecurities to direct your behavior, the best thing that can happen is the development of the relationship. In the worst-case scenario, you will learn to grow within yourself.

Simple Tips For Getting Rid Of Relationship Anxiety

Pistanthrophobia, also known as relationship anxiety, is something that almost

20% of people suffer from. It is the fear of blindly trusting new people who are introduced into your life. The fear, as we know, originates from the past experiences where you failed. The anxious thoughts, along with the concerns, can come as overwhelming waves. They are enough for reliving all the traumatizing events of your life that took place in the past. Relationship anxiety can spread its head in several ways. Your concern for your partner about what they are doing, testing your partner all the time for proving their love to you, or accusing them of not providing you with something that you need are some of the ways in which relationship anxiety might show up.

Now that you have gained enough knowledge about relationship anxiety and what it looks like, here are some tips that can help you cope with all your consuming thoughts.

- **Communicate:** Communication is a complicated topic, specifically for all those who are affected by anxiety. At times, people who suffer from anxiety might face some hard time expressing what they feel, and might also feel misunderstood. You might find it easier to run away from various situations that need addressing your anxiety level. However, make sure that you do not build up walls or push others away. You are required to be completely attuned with your partner and with yourself. Try not to shut down the situation. In case you still cannot cope up with the situations, try to let your partner know that the distance between you two is because of anxiety. Start communicating in case you need your space. Also, let your partner know when you want to talk to them. Your partner should also feel the urge to communicate back about the struggles they are facing as well.

- **Discovering your own self:** Even when you try to be your best and use up your full potential, you might not always reach your goal. There are very rare cases when we can reach out to our full potential. Your potential is the thing that you need to strive for continuously. It is more like a process and not a destination. Try to keep this in your mind and acknowledge that it is not possible to start all your relationships at your best all the time. Also, do not just search for a partner who will fill all the tender places of your life.

Self-discovery is an important aspect. It will permit you to listen to everything that is going on inside you. It will also help you to accept yourself the way you are. Slowly building up the confidence in your true self is the most effective way of overcoming anxiety. Keep in mind that the process related to self-discovery might turn out to be lengthy. So, it will not help you if you be impatient. In case you are unsure where to begin from, you can start by writing down all your unique aspects and talents. You can ask your partner to provide you with the required support for walking through this road.

- **Therapy:** If you are facing difficulty in finding your true self, opting for individual or even group therapy can help. It is a very effective way to start searching for understanding. As you speak up with a counselor, you will find it a lot easier to examine your shortcomings and struggles uniquely compared to a person you trust.

Therapy will not only be helping you to work through various kinds of stuff, but it can also provide you with the required tools for dealing with future stuff. When you verbalize all your feelings with a therapist, they can help you re-shape all your coping mechanisms. You will be able to lead to a better emotional life.

- **Changing your internal dialogue:** What you decide to pay attention to will shape your mentality and form your reality. Some people might also feel that they are the only victim of anxiety and just internalize his belief. However, there is a completely different way to perceive reality in a different way that will ultimately result in inner peace. The first step is to be aware of your inner sayings. You can start with meditation to be aware of your deep-seated thoughts. After you are aware of your thoughts, and in case you find that the thoughts are negative, try to think something positive purposefully. The second step is to practice living in the moment. Try to concentrate on all those things that are taking place around you.

- **Caring for yourself:** A very powerful and important management strategy is to take care of yourself. Apart from exercising and eating right, taking proper care of yourself also involves meditation, relaxation, enough sleep, maintaining a journal, and spending a happy time with friends and family. All of these are mere tools for managing your anxiety. If you start considering these as the cure, you are completely wrong. You will be able to bring a fundamental change in the way of your life.

- **Setting up boundaries:** Establishing the need and sense of limits and boundaries can help you get a clear picture of your feelings, needs, and decisions. As you build up boundaries, you will feel safe, relaxed, and empowered. In return, it will result in less anxiety and reduced compulsive behavior. You will need to alter your boundaries in case you:
1. Cannot say no
2. Avoid serious relationships
3. Face difficulty in communicating your feelings and needs
4. Are not sure about your feelings

If all of the above sounds quite familiar to you, there are several ways in which you can establish new boundaries. However, you will need to remeber that establishing boundaries takes time and can be tricky. If you opt for therapy, setting up boundaries would be a great goal. To set your limits and decide what is acceptable and what is not, you will need to gain knowledge about limits first. Try to figure out your intellectual and emotional limits concerning others. In case you are not sure, try to recall some of your past experiences that resulted in rage, anger, discomfort, or fatigue. Now, you can easily determine what your limits are in relation to your family members, friends, partner, or coworkers. As you consider the triggers from your past experiences, setting future boundaries will seem a lot easier.

- **Staying busy:** When you stay busy mentally, it can easily improve your relationship's overall mood. Often you will find that your thoughts and your mind are your biggest enemies. For example, you might just imagine having a fight with your partner. So, in such cases, you can try to keep your mind busy with other activities like reading books, watching TV, and others. This way, you can control your mind from traveling through negative paths.
- **Exercising and other strategies:** Anxiety, no matter of what type it is, it is still anxiety. So, it

can be said that effective strategies for the reduction of anxiety can help a lot in controlling the way you feel. One of the easiest strategies for coping up with anxiety is exercising. It has been found that exercise is much more effective in reducing anxiety than medications for anxiety control.

- **Starting over:** If you think the trust is gone, try to it discuss with your partner about the same. You can talk and start over the relationship as if both of you were never dating before. Trust is all about setting up a foundation. It is required to be grown from the ground level. Also, you must stick to it from the very beginning. After a few weeks, if you feel that the trust is back, it would be better to continue with the same. You would not like to return to old habits.

- **Exchanging one another's needs:** Try having a conversation with your partner regarding what you both need. You can also write them down in a journal so that it is known to both of you. After that, try your best to provide your partner with all they need. You can ask for the same in return from your partner, but make sure you do not hurt their morals. Sometimes, you might also find your partner willing to change themselves for the betterment of the relationship.

- **Try to be affectionate physically:** Holding hands and touching, even at times when you are angry at your partner, can turn out to be soothing. It is one of the prime reasons why most of the successful couples hug each other after returning home from work. Try your best to be more affectionate physically. It will send a relaxing reminder that you both will be together, no matter what happens.

Anxiety does not need to penetrate your relationship and mind forever. There are professionals and several other strategies that can help you in healing and reshaping your thinking process. In place of just being caught up in your thoughts, try to navigate the same towards positive, healthy actions, and thinking. Relationship anxiety might urge you to control your romantic partner's thoughts, actions, and basic whereabouts. But it is not possible. The only individual whom you can keep under your control is you.

So, whenever relationship anxiety hits you and you feel like jumping to conclusions, or just check the text messages of your partner, stop yourself. Try to consider the emotions and their point of origin mindfully. Take total control of the process and change the direction of the path. You will need to be patient with yourself during this practice. Coping with relationship anxiety involves sorting every layer of your thoughts and emotions. Always remember that these layers might run very deep at times. The best thing that can be done on your pat is to start the healing process by following the initial steps. Seek for help if required.

Chapter 5: Self-Evaluation Of Relationship Anxiety

How are you going to know that you are suffering from relationship anxiety? Are there any definite signs that can determine the various kinds of negative emotions regarding your relationship? How can anxiety affect your relationship? All such questions can be easily answered when you opt for what is known as self-evaluation of relationship anxiety. You will learn the basics of self-evaluation that can help in relieving tension from your relationship in this chapter. The aim of this is to properly evaluate the issue for putting a complete end to it.

Anxiety can crop up any time in relationships. The truth is that every one of us is vulnerable to this basic kind of problem. You will find that the tendency to get anxious in a healthy relationship will increase as the bond tends to grow stronger. So, everyone needs to opt for self-evaluation. Are you in the habit of spending most of your time worrying about all those things that could go bad in your relationship? A definite sign of relationship anxiety is when you keep worrying as an outcome of all the questions that run in your mind. For the perfect self-evaluation of this definite problem, you will first learn about the signs that will depict whether you are anxious or not. You will also require to assess the effects and causes of the problem that you think persists in your relationship. As already mentioned before, the cause of evaluation is to learn about the problems before they can develop.

How To Find Out You Are Suffering From Anxiety In Your Relationship?

You might be submerged in the deep sea of relationship anxiety without having any idea of it. In this section, you will find the symptoms of the problems related to you.

- **When you are jealous of your romantic partner:** Take a proper look at your normal behavior. Do you feel like breaking someone's face when your partner gets close to someone else of the opposite sex? Are you scared of any of your partner's friends who you think might rob your partner from you? You are suffering from jealousy if that is the case. It is one of the signs that you are suffering from relationship anxiety. At times, you might also feel like testing the love and commitment of your partner towards you. All of this is a clear indication of relationship anxiety sparked by jealousy.

- **When your self-esteem level tends to be low:** Do you always try to be cautious regarding how you behave in front of your partner? You might tend to do this because you are not sure how your partner will react. You are scared to express your true self in front of your partner because you fear rejection. It is a very clear indication of low self-esteem, which is also a sign of relationship anxiety.
- **Trust issues:** When you are in a healthy relationship, your partner should be the person whom you can trust the most. If you tend to confirm what your partner says right before you can believe them, it is an indication of trust issues in your relationship. Most of the time, lack of trust results from past betrayal. But you should never let your betrayals from the past to negatively impact your relationship. You will need to understand that no one is perfect in this world. Once your partner assures you that certain incidences will not happen again, try to believe them. A relationship will never work if you cannot blindly trust your partner.
- **Emotional imbalance:** You feel angry today, frustrated tomorrow, and happy the next day. It is known as emotional instability. You might

not have any clear idea about the same. However, continuous mood swings are also an indication of emotional imbalance. They are not going to help the matter in any way. They will be worsening it only. No matter what problems or tensions you are going through, try to talk about them with your romantic partner. When both partners try to work on a problem, the chances are high that the issue will get resolved very quickly. When you find out that you cannot stabilize your mood, it signifies relationship anxiety.

- **Reduced sex drive and lack of sleep:** The immediate result of constant worry is insomnia. You will be unable to have proper sleep. As you cannot sleep, you are most likely to feel stressed, resulting in decreased libido. All of these can also be regarded as a symptom of relationship anxiety.

In case you are experiencing any or all of these symptoms, you will need to determine its cause. Dealing with the causes of relationship anxiety is very important. Let's have a look at some of the causes of all these problems.

Probable Causes Of Relationship Anxiety

Majority of the time, relationship anxiety might turn out to be the manifestation of a problem that is rooted deep inside. Some of the most common causes are:

- **Relationship complication:** When the relationship is not defined clearly, or you are not certain about the same, it is classified as being complicated. It can be regarded to all those people who are in the dating stage. For example, a woman might not be clear about a man's motive – whether they are in the relationship just for fun or want to take it to marriage. Even long-distance relationships can lead to relationship anxiety. If this is the case, then both partners are required to trust each other.

- **Continuous fights:** When you just keep on fighting or quarreling with your partner, you will not be able to put an end to your worries. You will always feel tensed or worried as you are unsure when the next fight will crop up. It is a major cause of relationship anxiety. The reason behind this is that your intention of avoiding fights will not let you spend some quality time with your romantic partner.

- **Always comparing:** Comparison of the current relationship with the past ones needs to be avoided. It is not at all a healthy practice. You might breed in the feelings of intense regret in case you find out that the last relationship was far better in regards to communication, intimacy, finance, and various other aspects. To keep yourself away from such feelings, never compare your relationship or even marriage in regards to others or the ones from your past.

- **Less understanding:** Partners who do not want to invest time to understand one another are bound to suffer from difficulties. As already mentioned above, continuous fights will lead to relationship anxiety. Can you notice the anxiety symptoms along with miscommunications? When understanding is lacking between two partners, relationship anxiety will crop up. Try to invest some time to get to know your partner in a better way. Also, encourage your partner to do the same.

- **Miscellaneous issues:** Tough experiences from your past relationships can lead to other serious issues. Also, neglect or abuse in the past and lack of affection are some of the definite reasons you might suffer from relationship anxiety.

After you have successfully figured out the prime cause of the issues related to your relationship, getting rid of that cause is going to be the next big step. In the next section, we will discuss some of the steps for dealing with the issues' cause.

How To Get Rid Of The Root Cause?

Couples/partners are bound to face various types of challenges which they need to address as they progress. Your capability to manage the issues as they crop up in the relationship will help determine the relationship growth. In case a challenge or issue is not managed properly, you might find your healthy relationship in a phase of crisis. You might also need to take some serious steps to find your way out of the issue. Some of the most common challenges faced by people in their relationships are relationship needs, communication, developing jointly as a couple, equal rights, contentedness, habit, routine, loyalty, sexuality, fights, stress, value differences, conflicts, illness, distance, and this list will keep going on.

How much careful are you and your partner in the relationship? Being considerate and careful can help in avoiding most of the frustrations in your relationship. Are you able to enjoy the moment? Living in the present sounds much easier than doing the same. It might not be now, but sometimes our thoughts from the past or the future will try to slide in. There are certainly other questions that you will need to ask yourself. How much are you enjoying the present moment? Can you make your partner understand what you want to say? Do you both spend a lot of time together doing common things? Can you feel tenderness, sexual satisfaction, and security with your partner? Do you find support and peace in the relationship? Can you discuss anything openly with your partner? Do you feel strong with your partner?

As you answer all of these questions, you will be able to guide yourself properly in the road of self-evaluation of various issues that you are facing in the relationship. In most cases, men, in particular, do not like to get indulged in relationship talks. Regardless of that, it is important to regularly exchange your wishes and needs with your partner. Communication strategies play a vital role, especially for resolving conflicts. First, you will need to learn about distinguishing between general communication as partners and communication resulting from conflict resolution.

Communicating about each other's wishes, hopes, plans, and ideas forms an important foundation block of a relationship. Those couples who are happy for a long time in their relationships can communicate with each other about their feelings. They do not see the relationship or themselves being threatened by all their expressions. It won't even matter if both of them are negative about their feelings without having an idea about the same. They can develop their own gestures, facial expressions, and subtle language throughout the course of their relationship. Fights and quarrels are very normal in a healthy relationship. All that matters is the 'HOW.' Clashes tend to arise whenever you or the other person feels strained by various external stresses. For example, conflicts in the family, problems in raising children, problems in the job, and many others. The partner who feels stressed will communicate with the other person in a more violent or irritated tone.

It is always in your greatest interest to be inventive and proactive in relation to the way you communicate with all those who are closest to you. Creating, nurturing, and maintaining relationships with family, friends, and co-workers, not just our partners, is important for our well-being. Instead of just waiting for others to bring in changes in the relationships, the best and the easiest place for starting is with your own self.

Self-Assessment Of A Relationship

Below a list of certain statements have been provided that are very common in relationships. Try to check all the statements and note any of the statements that you feel like are not true for you. Write them down in a journal.

1. I can get on very well with all the siblings.
2. I have told my partner/children/spouse that I like them within a period of a few weeks or days.
3. I can be friendly with my clients or co-workers.
4. I can get on well with my employees.
5. There is no such person who can make me feel uncomfortable while walking across.
6. I have the habit of positioning relationships at first and results in second.
7. I have successfully destroyed all those relationships that tend to hurt me or injure me.
8. I have tried to communicate will all those people I might have injured, hurt, or disturbed.
9. I do not like or have the habit of gossiping about others.
10. I try to tell the truth all the time, even when I am hurt.
11. I have an effective circle of family or friends who I appreciate and love.
12. I get enough love from everyone around me for feeling appreciated.
13. I always try to stick to my word. Others can rely on me.

14. I always forgive all those people who hurt me.
15. I try my best to clear misunderstandings or miscommunications right after they take place.
16. I do not criticize or judge other people.
17. Nothing is unresolved concerning my past relationships.
18. I live my life completely based on my own terms. I do not base my life on the preferences or principles of other people.
19. I am aware of my desires and needs. I make sure others take care of them.
20. I have a lover or supporter.

Problem: Struggles Regarding Household Responsibilities

Most of the partners work at different places or, at times, more than a single job. So, it is very important to divide the responsibilities of the household fairly.

Strategies:

- Try to be clear and organized regarding your work or job in your home. You can write down all the roles and decide who is going to do what. It will be better for both partners if you can be clear about the things you do not want to do

and want to do. Make sure you figure out the time for all your jobs.
- It is always a good thing to be open to alternatives. If you do not like to take up the job of cleaning your house, you can opt for a cleaning service. In case you focus on being neat, but the other person does not, do you need to compromise? Always try your best for meeting right in the middle. Compromising will lead to future conflicts.

Problem: Money

There are various relationships in which the problems crop up from money. Whether there has been some sort of mistrust because of mismanagement of the finances, or one partner manages finances better than the other, money is capable of easily straining even the rock-solid relationships.

Strategies:

- Try to be honest in relation to the present financial scenario. It will be better for you if you do not opt for the topic in tense situations. You can always set a convenient and suitable time when you both can discuss the topic of finance.

- You will need to acknowledge that one of you will always be a saver while the other partner will be a spender. You will need to discuss the positive side of each. Try to learn as much as possible from one another.
- Do not ever hide your financial debts or gains from your partner. If both of you want to join your finances at some point of time, present all the financial documents along with pay stubs, insurance policies, credit reports, investments, bank statements, and debts.
- If anything goes wrong regarding finances, never try to blame your partner, even if they are at fault. The numbers on your computer screen and the paper pieces are not significant compared to your human bond and connection.
- When you opt for sharing your money, try to bring all your savings under a joint budget. Payout all the monthly bills from that joint budget. Both of you can still put aside some money for spending whenever needed.
- Making decisions about your short term and long term goals is very important. It is very normal to have your own goals. However, you should not also underestimate your family goals.

- It is a natural thing when one partner takes more financial responsibilities than the other. In such cases, never try to undermine your partner if you are the one who takes more responsibilities.

Problem: Not Keeping The Relationship On The Priority List

If you are willing to maintain the relationship and want to keep it healthy, prioritizing is very important. Try to understand its importance. Try to cherish your relationship and nourish the same. This way, you can stand out with your partner in the relationship in the test of time.

Strategies:

- Start doing all those things that you used to do during the initial days of the relationship. It is said that the starting days of a relationship are always the most soothing ones. Give compliments to each other, appreciate each other, communicate with each other throughout the day, and showcase genuine interest in one another.
- Try to take out some time from the busy schedule and go on a date. Make every effort to plan the date with the level of consideration, just like

you both were trying to win over each other during the initial days.
- Always keep in mind that respect is a very important component of a healthy relationship. In case you cannot appreciate someone much, learn to do that. When your partner tries to do something that genuinely makes you smile or happy, do not hesitate to show the gratitude by simply saying thank you. Just let your partner understand what are the things that matter to you and them.

Problem: Conflicts

Occasional fights and conflicts are very natural and are more or less a part of our lives. But in case you and your partner keep arguing all the time, the time has come to break the cycle. You both need to get freed from such a poisonous routine. In place of just igniting your anger, try to look closely into the underlying problems. Try to find out how you can solve the problem without any risk of hostility.

Solution:

- Both of you will need to argue in a useful and civil manner. It can help in suppressing the fire of conflict.

- You will need to realize that you are not the victim. It is perfectly your choice for reacting the way you do. Try to be honest with yourself along with your partner regarding how you truly feel.
- Once you are in the center of a heated argument, try to pay attention to how you phrase things along with the voice tone. Will you be feeling okay if your partner also spoke to you in the same way, in the same tone? You will need to put kindness and love first. Never forget that the individual you are arguing with is also the person you have chosen to be your life partner. Do you find the conflict of more worth than your relationship? Try to respect the relationship along with your partner, even while arguing. If you want to prove a point, just stay calm and explain yourself to your partner with a soothing tone and not something violent.
- If you keep on responding with a similar kind of approach that already invited unhappiness and pain in your life, it will be foolish of you if you expect something different. For instance, if you have the habit of stopping your partner in the middle while they talk just because you are willing to defend yourself, stop doing that for some

time. You will feel amazed and shocked after seeing how much a tempo change can affect your argument tone.

- Do not hesitate to apologize to your partner when you realize that you are the one who is wrong. It is a great way in which you can show your partner that you respect their values much ahead of being right. Just give this is a try and see the results.

- You can never manage or control the behavior of someone else. You need to remember that the only person whom you can control is yourself. So, when you try to shift your focus from your partner's behavior and concentrate on yours, you will find it easier to resolve any conflict.

Problem: Trust

Trust is very important as far as a healthy relationship is concerned. Are you concentrating on all those things that might make your trust for your romantic partner fade away? Are you having certain issues that are not resolved yet and are making it tough for you to trust your partner? If that is the case, you will need to work on the same as soon as possible. Whenever trust issues crop up in a relationship, the chances are high that it will weaken the relationship's foundation if not taken care of properly.

Strategies:

You can develop trust in your partner and vice versa if both of you try to consider the mentioned pointers.

- Try to be punctual.
- Try not to be inconsistent.
- Try being fair, even while arguing.
- Never fail from doing all that you have promised.
- Stop yourself from lying, no matter what the situation is.
- Call up when you have that you will.
- Try being sensitive to the feelings of your partner. You might still disagree with your partner but do not undermine his/her feelings.
- Let your partner know whenever you will be reaching home late.
- Try to carry your weight. Fulfill all your responsibilities and promises.
- Always keep yourself away from hurting the old wounds.
- Try not to say those things that you can never take back.

- Prevent yourself from being jealous without any need.
- Have respect for the boundaries of your partner.
- Try to be realistic. When you just think that your romantic partner will be able to meet all your needs and wants, while you expect them to understand everything without expressing what you need, it can be treated as a fantasy from a Hollywood movie. Just ask your partner for all that you need and do not just expect them to read your mind.

You are always required to be all ready for making the relationship work from all positive sides. Try to look into those things that need to be done for keeping up the healthy state of the relationship. Do not just come to the conclusion that you cannot maintain a loving and peaceful relationship with your partner until and unless you give a look over the conflicts. Make sure you address them all. If you fail to attend to all the active issues in your relationship, your relationship will be marred with all of these problems.

Chapter 6: Identifying Various Behaviors That Can Trigger Anxiety

Anxiety is always regarded as an unhealthy thing, and it can easily impart a huge impact on our lives. It can easily stop you from doing all those things that you need or desire. As you feel anxious, you might feel that some external forces are controlling your entire life. Anxiety takes the form of a vicious and negative cycle that is powerful enough for consuming you completely. It can affect your hobbies, relationship, well-being, and many more. It might feel a lot tough to break open from the cycle of anxiety. However, there is still some possibility. Anxiety can make you feel that you have lost all control over your life and cannot even do anything regarding the same. But you can also learn to keep your anxieties under control and seek for happiness.

Anxiety disorder crops up when you feel inappropriate levels of tension, worry, or fear resulting from certain emotional triggers regularly. The ability to identify the various reasons that are leading to your anxiety attacks is the only key to a successful treatment.

- **Genetics:** It has been found that anxiety disorder might turn out to be genetic. In simple terms, if any of your family members suffered from an anxiety disorder, the chances are high that you will experience the same at some point in your life.
- **Environmental factors:** All the elements that are present around you can also trigger anxiety. Stress and worries that are linked to a relationship, school, monetary problems, or job can result in anxiety disorder.
- **Medical factors:** There are various medical issues that can trigger anxiety disorder. For example, drug side effects, stress from medical conditions, or symptoms of illness. All such conditions can result in certain lifestyle changes such as restricted movement, pain, and also emotional imbalance.
- **Brain chemistry:** All those experiences that are stressful and traumatizing can easily affect the performance and structure of your brain. It can force the brain to react vigorously to certain triggers that might not have resulted in anxiety before.

Relationships are always considered to be very fulfilling. A healthy relationship can help in filling up the vacuum of your life. It can provide you with opportunities for fun, happiness, exciting dates, interesting conversations, and, most importantly, love. However, all these might also turn out to be the sources of worry and upheaval. Your capability to identify the prime sources of relationship anxiety can help you maintain a distance from them. Thus, it can enhance the stability and balance of the relationship. Now, I will discuss some of the most common relationship anxiety triggers and how you can control them.

What can trigger relationship anxiety the most? It is right when you are extremely vulnerable to someone else. We search for love and safety in a healthy relationship. If you have the experience of getting hurt before, the fear of the same can trigger your current relationship anxiety. The financial concern of both partners in a relationship is one more cause that can trigger anxiety. Majority of the time, people try not to disclose their issues related to finances fully. They tend to open up and discuss only when they face something serious. However, by this point of time, it might turn out to be too late. It might be that you are not at all compatible with the other person about expenditure and saving money, or the money views of both of you do not even match. Whenever real-life expenditures come in the picture, and you just move around with the burden of the same, anxiety tends to set in. Money is a constant in almost all relationships.

The fear of rejection, along with being abandoned, can also trigger anxiety. The insecurities that you possess are reflected back to you by your romantic partner. It is a normal thing to worry about such things. However, instead of just piling them inside yourself, it is always better to speak up about them. Try to discuss the insecurities that you suffer from with your partner. You are required to create a stronger sense of yourself. You need to learn how to be aware of your thought process and state of mind all the time to keep anxieties out of the way. The arguments that you mostly have with your partner over your work, money, social life, or family comes with some sort of rejection as the roots. The deep-seated fear and feeling of such fights are that you might get abandoned. For example, if you are having an argument with your partner about the amount of time they spend with their family or friends, it is all about why your partner is not spending the same time with you.

As you improve your ability to stay relaxed in the relationship, it can help to make you feel less rejected and less defensive. Try to be present by yourself in the relationship and remove all sorts of negative thoughts. You are required to set up definite boundaries regarding the information type that you allow in your head. Keep working for preventing unwanted behaviors and information from entering and penetrating your thoughts. Whenever you feel like anxiety is knocking at the door, just open up the door for it. Try to address the anxiety, give it a look, take a deep breath, and then close the door. There is no need to welcome your anxieties all the time with open arms. However, you can acknowledge that it is present.

Definite Triggers Of Anxiety

When you keep contacting your ex, it can easily trigger relationship anxiety. You must handle communications with your ex very cautiously. The primary reason behind this is that it can result in anger, anxiety, and slowly a sudden breakup in the current relationship. In case you have to still maintain the communication with your ex, explain to your partner the reason behind the same. Make sure the communication is transparent and platonic. If there is no need to communicate your ex, just don't do it. It can effectively hamper your present relationship and will lead to anxiety.

Distance, coupled with a lack of communication, can also contribute to relationship anxiety between partners. Whenever you do not get your partner's physical availability for a long time, you might find it tough to get the required assurance. As a result, anxiety will crop up. Even when you communicate with your partner over the phone and on video calls daily, you might still feel the void deep in your heart. In such situations, you are required to depend only on the power of words as you communicate all your feelings with your romantic partner. Just feel free while expressing your partner your requirements from them. Try to discuss about insecurities, if any. As you do so, you will provide your partner with the ability to assure you of their commitment and love.

Another definite trigger of anxiety in a relationship is doubt. It might lead you to question every action and move of the other person, thinking whether you took the right decision or what steps you need to take next. In case you find yourself in great doubt, start making some conscious efforts to release yourself from the doubts. Divert your mind from all those questions that are making you doubt your partner or the relationship. Just inhale deeply and calm yourself down. Allow your mind to enjoy the road of relationship. Provide all the freedom to your partner and also to your mind. Stop yourself from making any decisions concerning the relationship for some time.

How To Put An End To Such Behaviors?

Anxiety will not only make you feel stressed, but it can also distress the relationship. Staying in a relationship where the other person in anxious might be very confusing. So, you must take some serious steps to address the triggers of the same. Also, note that the experiences and quality of a relationship can result in anxiety. It is not required to be necessarily about the behavior or attitude of your partner. As you grow in the relationship, things might turn out to get complicated. Keeping your anxiety in control in a relationship has more to do with yourself compared to your partner.

The most useful way of putting an end to your anxieties and its triggers in the relationship is by exercising and practicing other strategies for anxiety reduction. It has been found that daily exercising can help in relieving stress and anxiety to a great extent. You can also opt for rebuilding the relationship trust as a clear way of wiping out all anxieties that might exist. Starting your relationship from the beginning can also help. Trust and relationship grow side by side. Provide some time to your partner and yourself for cultivating a trusting and loving relationship once more. Communication also plays an important role in quenching all your anxieties. If you cannot remember your desires and needs, write them down. Readout loud to your partner all your needs and desires. Transparency is the only way of sustaining a healthy relationship. Also, make sure that you address the desires and needs of your partner with the same dedication.

Another useful way of preventing your anxious behaviors is by being busy mentally. As you fill up your thoughts and mind with other activities and concerns of productive nature, you can easily divert your mind from the relationship's anxious thoughts. It will ultimately reduce the frequency in which you allow your mind to wander into the arena of negative thoughts and emotions. Productive activities like reading books, going out on dates, spending time with friends, watching movies, and opting for outdoor activities can improve your relationship mood. Try to be physical with your partner, as much as you can, during moments of anxiety. Hold hands, touch your partner, and kiss them when you feel mad at them. Staying affectionate even during times of difficulty or stress can help the partners to reconnect with each other. It will also assure that the intimacy and love in the relationship have not yet vanished.

You will have to keep putting efforts from your side. Learn how to calm yourself down, comfort yourself, and reassure yourself in situations of anxiety. Deep breathing exercises can help a lot in dealing with anxious situations. You will be able to manage issues of panic, calm down, and reduce your levels of stress. As you keep breathing deeply, you will shift all your concentration on the process of breathing. The process involves your rib cage and belly being completely filled with every inhalation, along with complete exhalations. Such easy breathing exercises can help in reducing stress and anxiety drastically. You will tend to feel more energized, refreshed, and relaxed. As you take full breaths, you will be able to calm yourself down and keep the control in your hand as anxiety keeps knocking on the door.

Every relationship requires tenderness, trust, a touch of vulnerability, and patience. Individuals who suffer from anxiety generally comes with plenty of all these. They are also capable of providing all these to the relationship connection liberally. The main problem is that the anxious thoughts work in full fledge for eroding most of the qualities. Relationships are bound to face struggles. However, once anxiety comes into play, it tends to amplify the struggles and make them tough to manage.

An Effective Breathing Exercise

While practicing this breathing exercise, you must be in a calm environment with pin-drop silence before you can move to the next steps. Start by sitting in a chair upright. You can also opt for sitting on the floor in any position in which you feel comfortable. Shut your eyes for reflecting all your concentration inwards and focus. Start being aware of your breathing pattern. Is the breathing pattern very fast or slow? Now start breathing intentionally. Ensure that your shoulders are relaxed, and you are sitting still. Start inhaling slowly and deeply through your nostrils. You can feel that the diaphragm is expanding as fill the body with air. Start exhaling the inhaled air slowly through your mouth. It will allow you to remove the stale air from the body.

Keep on focusing on your pattern of breath for five to ten cycles. The moment you start with the breathing exercise, you will see that certain areas of the body are already feeling less tense than the other areas. The reason behind this is that the body starts releasing stress as you exhale. Right before you stop this exercise, make sure you notice how you feel emotionally, mentally, and physically. For getting the most from this exercise, you will need to practice this exercise daily. You can also practice this exercise at any time when you start feeling anxious.

Another great strategy that can help you in coping up with anxiety is the exercise of progressive muscle relaxation. The muscle relaxation exercise is very helpful for reducing the disturbing bouts that come with anxiety. It is a relaxation technique and can help you very much at times of panic attack or during high stress. As you relax your body, you can let go of all the anxious feelings and thoughts.

Step-By-Step Technique: Progressive Muscle Relaxation

Begin by being in a comfortable position. You can lie down or sit down. Get rid of all kinds of distractions. Close your eyes for better concentration. Start breathing deeply through your nose. You can feel your abdomen rise up as you fill up air in the body. Exhale slowly from your mouth, draw your navel in the direction of your spine. Keep doing this for four to five times. Tighten the muscles of your feet, followed by relaxation of the same muscles. Clench your toes, press the heels in the direction of the ground. The aim is to squeeze your body's muscles for a few breaths, followed by releasing the muscles. Keep tightening and releasing each group of muscles. Bring into action the muscles of your arms, hands, legs, neck, face, shoulders. End the exercise by inhaling a few more breaths. You will find that your muscles are relaxed. It will help in ultimately calming you down at times of excessive anxiety.

How To Put An End To Your Worries?

As you deal with panic or anxiety disorder, worry will always be in a commonplace. You feel worried about the relationship state, your partner, your future, your finances – the list keeps going on. You might also find yourself getting worried about all those things that never happened or are not within your control. For example, safety, health, relationship security, and many other issues that keep draining you. As you keep worrying, it will eventually take the shape of a burden. It is powerful enough to affect a healthy relationship in a negative way. It can also affect your self-esteem, personality, career, and several other life aspects. You might also find yourself breaking down mentally and emotionally. So, it is beneficial to know how you can put all your worries at bay. There is no need to allow your worries to control the pace of your life. It can be reduced effectively by taking some important steps.

- Fix a time to think about your worries. It might seem counterintuitive for scheduling a worrying time. However, this might turn out to be all that you need for dealing with your anxious thoughts. Start by determining the time of day that you want to put aside for worrying. You can fix the time in the morning so that it gets easier for you to get rid of your worries and spend the rest of the day on a happy note. It can be during the night as well so that you can let go of your worries right before you go to sleep. It is very effective in clearing up the worries in your mind that keep piling up during the day.
- Discuss with others about your worries. You might find some immediate relief as you share all your feelings and thoughts with a family member or a close friend. Family members can always turn out to be one of the greatest supports. You can get all the support and love that you need from them. They can even provide you with proper guidance throughout this period.

- Keeping a journal for working through all your anxieties and worries is another useful way. If you think that you have no one to share your feelings or talk to, start maintaining a journal. Write down all your inner feelings, worries, and emotions. Read them every day and keep ticking them off as you successfully get rid of them.
- The act of positive thinking can help you to put a permanent stop to all your worries. Worry is nothing but a pattern of negative thinking. It can easily contribute to panic disorder and anxiety. Try to change all your thoughts' direction by concentrating on either side of the negative thoughts or worries. Make every effort to replace all your negative thoughts with positive and realistic statements.

Ways Of Working Through Your Worries

You might find it impossible all the time to put an end to your worries. However, there are some ways that can help you easily manipulate all your feelings that tend to take control over your life. At times, the perfect way of controlling your worries is by acknowledging them and then taking steps to reduce the same.

Getting Enough Sleep

After a day of heavy work or party, sometimes sleeping it off is the best remedy for feeling fresh and energetic. Anxiety and worry will tend to get more hold of you if you are physically and mentally exhausted. As you get enough sleep, you take the initiative to start solving the problems before they even start. Worry and anxiety are powerful enough for keeping us awake throughout the night. Even they can wake us up suddenly from our peaceful dreams. So, start taking advantage of your day naps for maintaining your levels of energy. Start working on your ability to push back worry. Whenever you get some free time, try to get some sleep. It can help to make you healthier, less irritable, and more concentrated in your work and personal life. It will ultimately be taking away most of the causes of your anxiety and worry, for example, poor performance at work or poor health.

Writing It Down

Journaling, as already mentioned before, is a useful way of dealing with worries and anxiety. Whenever you find that you are getting overwhelmed with your thoughts and cannot focus on anything, just write them down. Emptying your mind of all the thoughts and worries and putting them on paper can help. Sometimes, having a look at your worries and fears as you write them down can help you see how irrational or insignificant they are in real.

Following The Road Of Your Thoughts

It might feel like counterproductive as you concentrate on all those things that you worry about. However, sometimes it can help in playing out the fears in our minds. It can help discover that the end result you always think of might not turn out to be that bad at the end. So, whenever you feel like worrying, just follow your thoughts wherever they take you. For example, if you worry that your partner might get bored of you, try to play out all the consequences in your thoughts. If my partner is bored with me, they will look for some other person. If they search for someone else, they will succeed very easily as they are great. My partner will either cheat on me or will leave me for that other person. What next?

As you reach the endpoint of your thinking process, you can now closely examine all the event chains to determine how likely they are or what steps can be taken to prevent your partner from leaving you. For instance, you can return to the first thought of "my partner is bored of me" and think of ways in which you can spice up the relationship. No matter what is the reality, whether your partner is bored of you or not, it does not matter. If you can successfully acknowledge all your worries and fears and take the necessary steps for acknowledging them, you can remove the cause very easily. You can also remove the related symptoms.

Picking Up Something That Can Be Controlled

As mentioned in the last example, if you keep worrying about certain thoughts that can be acted upon, just do it. Most of your worry and anxiety originates from places of fears that make you believe that the 'unknown' is uncomfortable and scary. So, you must control the same so that you are aware of all those things you can expect. While it is true that you cannot come to know everything all the time, but you can take certain steps for preparing yourself against all those things that might come. There is no need to control your destiny. Just let things be in the way they are. Just take back your feeling of control by exerting certain influences.

Chapter 7: Relationship Conflicts

Conflicts are bound to crop up in relationships at any point of time. It could arise from financial problems, your career, your families who try to interfere in your relationship decisions, your new life with your baby, or your children's education. All such elements and some more are, most of the time, the major source of arguments that takes place between two partners. It can thus result in relationship conflicts. When such things happen, just try not to worry much. Arguments, at times, can bring out something good in the relationship. However, you should never allow negative situations or events to last for too long. If not taken care of, it can certainly weaken your relationship to a great extent. Relationship conflicts can be regarded as synonymous with the initial step that tends to destabilize a healthy relationship.

So, you will need to manage such situations properly for finding complicity, serenity, and last but not least, to revive the relationship flame. To make sure that the relationship can still continue or resume with a good start, you cannot allow things to worsen. You will be harming the relationship if you just stand idle and keep thinking that it will be better the next day. Love does not come up like that. You are required to keep working on your relationship and yourself. In case you fail to respond in time and just let a fight be in its place in your relationship, you will be risking the relationship to separation.

Primary Reasons For Relationship Conflicts

For facing the greatest monster in the relationship and the fears, the primary step is to learn about the origin of conflicts between you and your partner. Unless and until you get to know the origin, you will never be able to fix the issues properly. Putting your finger on the exact point of origin is of prime importance. For solving a problem in the best way, you are required to know the roots. Otherwise, you will end up putting a band-aid on the wound. Minute tensions can slowly take the shape of a big fight if you keep the relationship issues unresolved.

The first step for getting rid of relationship conflicts is to recognize them and then acknowledge the same. As already mentioned before, there might be several issues for the current situation of your relationship. Here are some of the primary reasons.

Conflicts Rising From Professional Life

Tensions are bound to arise in cases when you start caring more about your professional career compared to your partner. It works for your partner, as well. Such a situation can force you or your partner to react harshly. Nothing can feel worse than the feeling of being abandoned by the person you love. Concentrating on your professional life more than your personal life might not only turn out to be unhealthy when you are not in a relationship. It can show various adverse effects and destroy a healthy relationship. It might turn out to be very tough to reconcile family and work sometimes, specifically when you want to start with a new business or sustain a very stressful job. However, to have a balanced life and avoid relationship conflicts, you must learn how to disconnect yourself from work and enjoy your life with all those you love. However, to have a balanced life and avoid relationship conflicts, you must learn how to disconnect yourself from work and enjoy your life with all those you love.

Inappropriate Behavior And Infidelity

Certain attitudes need to be ground as you are in a relationship. If you keep sticking to a certain behavior that is considered to be unforgivable by your partner, you find it difficult to pick up the broken pieces. You will be pushing your relationship to some serious periods of turbulence. There might also be some serious conflicts between both partners in case of infidelity. If you find yourself in this kind of situation, you might face struggles beyond this book's capacity. Opt for therapy, either for yourself or for both partners.

When One Partner Fails To Meet The Expectation Of The Other

Life is bound to evolve, grow, and change. Relationships also pass through the same stages. At times, partners in a relationship tend to grow out separately. They reach a certain point where they are not the people they were during the relationship's starting days. Whenever such a thing happens, just sit down with your partner and discuss the same. What are all those expectations that either or both of you have that are not being met successfully? Are all those expectations reasonable? The best way to determine the condition and position of the relationship is by talking about it.

To overcome the major conflicts in your love life, no matter where the tensions originate from, the primary thing that you must do is understand why the fights and conflicts are there for starting with. To achieve this, try talking to your partner. You might find the discussion to be very uncomfortable, but it is required. Your anxiety levels might get heightened, but do not allow them to push you towards harsh behaviors. Controlled and calm discussions can help you more for dealing with conflicts rather than arguments filled with anxiety. Most couples try to run away from conflicts as much as possible. The reason is very obvious; to keep tensions out of the relationship. Some couples keep blaming each other for being the reason for the arguments. Such reactions are not going to resolve the struggles. In turn, they might exacerbate the issues.

Struggles are common parts of relationships and life. Whenever they get ignored, they will start causing harm. When faced right on their face, they turn into those tools that can help couples grow in a relationship by resolving the conflicts hand in hand. Struggles can also crop up from various wrong assumptions about:

- Relationship and its nature
- Different assumptions about how certain things are required to be done around your house
- Job and work
- Different obligations of the partners
- Differences in values, wants, needs, or morals
- Poor form of communication

How To Deal With Relationship Conflicts?

If you have ever been in a healthy romantic relationship, you will know that fights and disagreements are inevitable. When two individuals decide to spend the majority of their time together, with their interests and lives intertwined, no one can stop them from disagreeing. Such disagreements can either be small or big, ranging from whether one partner should move for the career of the other, what to have for dinner, or deciding about children's upbringing. The fact is that fighting with your partner is not a real sign of trouble in the relationship. When handled in the right away, conflicts can help in improving the chore of the relationship. If two partners never talk about their problems and fight over something, reaching a common ground will be tough. As you start dealing with your relationship conflicts constructively, you will be able to understand your partner in a better way.

Resolving conflicts will allow both the partners to reach a solution that will work for both of them. However, if you fail to notice the issues and conflicts, they might escalate very quickly and lead to greater conflicts without resolving the primary issues. Any kind of conflict with your partner can easily make you feel weak, vulnerable, threatened, or attacked. It can even make you retreat and recoil. If you opt for the silent treatment whenever you feel let down by your partner, it will harm the relationship more than doing any good. The ultimate result will be breaking up of the relationship. The way you both choose to resolve conflicts can help determine whether your relationship is healthy or unhealthy.

Smoothing over, fighting, or denial can never be treated as long-term solutions. All that these can do is to act as a band-aid for covering the cracks in the relationship, which will eventually burst open. The key to a successful relationship is, therefore, to move beyond these three to compromise, or for the best of all, settlement or collaboration. If you and your partner decide upon compromising, both of you will need to give up on something for reaching a mid-point solution. It is somewhat better than lose/win but is not win/win. As you decide to collaborate, both of you will work together to create a win/win situation. Certain strategies can provide you with long-term solutions from conflicts.

<u>Examining Your Focus</u>

A conflict will take a harmful shape when you just focus on defense from the attacks in place of resolving the problems. Simply by focusing on all your suffering and pain, you will ensure that you keep experiencing the same. It is because where you focus on, all your energy will flow in that direction only. Our focus helps in determining the direction of our lives. If you are not willing to hit the pole, you will need to concentrate on what you want: to stay on the road. As you change the focus, you can effectively change all the results.

If you concentrate on where you do not want the relationship to head to, fighting, and allowing anger to build up, you can find yourself where you are not willing to be. This way, you will end up either in an unfulfilling and painful relationship or simply separated from your romantic partner. When you concentrate on resolving the conflicts together, you will be able to get all those outcomes that you want.

Turning Conflicts Into Great Opportunities

Do not try to get defensive, do not focus on winning, and do not keep on hammering your point. Why would someone want to lose their partner whom they love? As you learn that there are no losers in the game of love, you will learn to shift your focus from petty arguments. In this way, you can also establish a healthy form of communication. Conflicts are opportunities in disguise, opportunities for the couples to align their beliefs and outcomes. Conflicts are the chances for appreciating, understanding, and embracing the differences. Try to place yourself in the shoes of your partner. Make every effort to understand the experience of your partner. These emotions and experiences might turn out to be very uncomfortable. But if you keep on opting for comfort, you can never learn to grow.

Conflicts can provide you with the opportunity to get to know more about your partner. You can learn to love your partner deeply. Try and learn to view conflicts as simple transitions to better things, instead of reasons for a retreat. The next time you find yourself fighting and disagreeing with your partner and wonder how you can save the relationship, just focus on the relationship's positive side. Shift your focus from the negative aspects to the positive ones of the relationship. Decide together actively how to work towards a stronger and stable future.

Using Humor

If you find your relationship and yourself in a vindictive cycle, a great way to break the pattern is to use humor. Humor is very effective in releasing tension. It will let you and your partner concentrate on all those things that you both want. Learning various ways to save the relationship is better than arguing what both of you do not want, ultimately leading to another argument. In case you feel that an argument is escalating, take some time to derail the same. Try to argue with a humorous tone. You can also sing a funny song while arguing that can make your partner laugh. The aim is to make the conflict look ridiculous. When you both laugh together, you can make the base of the relationship stronger.

Starting an argument is very easy, but having the ability to use humor and reverse the cycle of argument is something that can help a relationship prosper. You can even crack lame jokes every time you think an argument is cropping up.

Practicing Acceptance

No one in this world is perfect. Our partners have habits or do certain things that tend to annoy us. In place of just thinking about your partner's bad habits or negative traits, try to concentrate on all those things that they can present in the table. Try to think about your partner's qualities that you love and how they can make you feel. You soon notice that you can divert your mind from all those things that made you feel crazy about your partner. It is all about a person whom you adore and love. There is no need to regard the negative things as the only qualities of your partner. You will need to put some energy into understanding the flaws of each other. You and your partner are the supporting pillars of your relationship. You need to support your partner whenever they need you and vice versa. Just communicate with each other. Assess the needs of each other and resolve issues in a fun way instead of just arguing.

Make efforts to understand the reason behind certain behaviors of your partner or what they want to say. Make every effort to understand what your partner feels. Also, you will need to be acceptable to yourself. Try to be honest with all your emotions and feelings. Just be your true self. Every individual comes with personal flaws. All those flaws can never be the reason why you are asking for help to save the relationship. When you love a person, you will need to love their flaws too. Just accept the way they are. If the flaws feel threatening for the relationship, discuss it over.

Working On Forgiveness

If you are looking out for ways by which you can save the relationship as your trust is broken, it is very natural for you to feel bitter, angry, mistrustful, hurt, along with a bunch of other negative emotions. If you are the one who is guilty and broke the trust, you are bound to feel ashamed. You might even want to justify all your actions or just blame the other person for everything. In such situations, it is required for both the partners to start working on forgiveness. It is not possible to just wake up in the morning and start feeling forgiving towards your romantic partner magically. Forgiveness cannot be attained easily. It is a long process. It involves a series of several small acts – practicing complete honesty, admitting all mistakes, and always putting your partner first – that needs time.

Forgiveness takes up several works. If you are responsible for breaking your partner's trust, you are bound to take responsibility. Try to be respectful of the way your partner felt hurt and provide them with the required space. Just place your partner first, and prevent yourself from getting into the vicious cycle of self-blame. If your partner breaks your trust, ask for some space, but do not stop communicating. Always let your partner be aware of the things that you will need for rebuilding the trust. The aim is to never give up.

Communication

You are enjoying a cup of coffee in a café. You see two couples sitting next to you. The couple who are sitting on the left starts arguing whether they should go for dinner with friends or not. One of the partners says, "It is never fun with them; you only said this the last time." The other partner replies, "You always keep saying that, as they are my friends. You never give a chance to my friends." The other partner gets angry and says, "Now, you will start adding to your own story." Both partners turn away from each other. They are just sitting in silence.

The couple who are sitting on your right is also discussing about going out with friends. One of the partners says, "I think it will go on for a few hours. It might not be that much fun, I think. What do you say?" The other partner says, "I surely get that. I want to go, but maybe we should just turn it down this time. Besides, it will be great if we could reach home early." Both the partners smile, kisses, and continue gossiping as they drink their coffee.

Both the couples who were present in front of you were going through a similar nature of conflict. To be precise, it was the same conflict. However, one of the couples knew how they could resolve their conflict, whereas the other did not have any idea of it. The first couple simply reacted by depending on their bad habits. The conflict successfully widened the gap between them. The second couple successfully used the conflict as a chance or opportunity for communicating their feelings to each other. It is the way how a relationship should be. Which of the couples you think was successful in fulfilling their relationship? Which of the two relationships you think is going to last longer? Communication always comes first in the list of how you are going to save your relationship. It is one of the perfect ways of resolving conflicts. The more you can communicate in a relationship, the more it is going to last.

<u>Asking Right Questions</u>

If you are looking for ways how to save your relationship, the chances are high that something has been wrong in your relationship for a long time. You are not only required to dig into the past for uncovering deeper and real issues, but also focus on the future. It all depends on asking yourself the perfect questions. First, make sure that you are starting this exercise with the right mindset. The aim is not to dig up old issues, place blames, or just tell your partner all their flaws or mistakes. You are required to bring some change in your mindset for introducing acceptance and gratitude. Try to embrace the fact that life is not happening to you, but for you. Even you can get the opportunity to grow and learn from the current relationship state, as long as you are open to all those things that your relationship wants to tell you.

Now you are all set to ask yourself some essential questions: What was the reason for your breakup? Are there any limiting beliefs that both of you have been living by that ultimately affected the course of the relationship? Is there any possibility to overcome them? What are the things that you want from your relationship in the future? What will be the prime focus of your relationship? Answering some or each of these questions can help you change the scenario of your relationship. It can assist you in resolving all the existing conflicts in no time.

Making Time For Touch

When you keep fighting with your partner all the time, when everything in the relationship tends to annoy you, being affectionate might turn out to be a tough job. However, you are required to make some time for touch. Touch and being affectionate does not always mean sex. It also includes sneaking a cozy morning hug before going to work, cuddling and watching a movie together on the couch, holding hands without any definite reason or while crossing the road, etc. There is a definite reason that makes you instantly feel good as you touch your partner. Hugging, cuddling, or even holding hands helps in releasing oxytocin. Oxytocin is a feel-good hormone in the brain that makes us feel loved and safe. It can help lower down stress, make us feel more connected with our partner, help sleep, and reduce blood pressure. You can all these benefits simply by reaching your partner and holding their hand in yours.

Do not ever withhold your physical affection in the relationship, even when you are super mad at your partner. In case you cannot do so, you will end up in an affectionless relationship. If you are willing to save your relationship, begin with physical touch. Try to cuddle with your partner before you sleep. Hold hands in front of everyone on the road or sneak a sudden kiss as you both prepare dinner in the kitchen. Physical affection is not the result of a happy and happening relationship. It creates a happening and happy relationship.

Try Being Direct

Sometimes people opt for not to come up and directly state all those things that are bothering them. It is a common thing in relationships, especially the ones where conflicts arise now and then. Instead of opting for the direct path, partners choose indirect ways to express all their displeasure. One of the partners might opt for speaking to the other partner in an arrogant way that implies underlying hostility. At times, partners might decide not to pay attention to the issues or just switch the topics when any issue crops up. Expressing your anger using such indirect ways cannot be regarded as constructive. You will not provide your partner, who is the prime target of all your negative behaviors, with a clear idea of how they should respond. When you are irritated, your partner knows it very well. However, when there is a lack of directness, it will leave your partner without direction or guidance about what they need to do to resolve the problem.

Learn To Talk About Your Feelings Without Putting Blames On Your Partner

All those statements made by you that seem to directly assault your partner's character can turn out to be harmful to the relationship. When a man who is frustrated by his partner's jealousy says, "You are completely irrational!" is inviting his partner for becoming more defensive. It might also lead to the shutting down of future conversations. A constructive strategy for dealing with such situations is to put into use "I statements," coupled with "behavioral descriptions." The "I statements" will focus on your feelings, without playing the blame game with your partner. The "behavioral descriptions" will focus on a particular behavior that you feel your partner is engaging in. It effectively shifts the focus from a character flaw. For example, the man in the above example can say, "I feel irritated when you say that I am flirting with someone else even during simple conversations."

Such tactics are of direct nature that does not play with the character of your partner.

However, you must note that all these direct tactics might turn out to be constrictive in certain situations. It has been found from studies that partners who have minor issues in their relationship, rejecting and blaming each other during a fight, can directly lower down the satisfaction in the relationship. It can also make the issues look worse than before. For all those couples who have major relationship issues, rejecting and blaming behaviors results in conflict discussion. With time, the issues will get resolved, leading to improved satisfaction in the relationship.

Never Saying 'Never' or 'Always'

When you opt for addressing a serious problem, try not to make generalizations regarding your partner. For example, "You never help me with the household works," or, "You are always busy with your phone." Such statements are most likely to turn your partner defensive. Instead of starting a conversation or discussion regarding how your partner can be more attentive or helpful, such statements can make them do the opposite. You will never want your partner to be defensive, right? So, instead of using 'never' or 'always' in your statements, try to use words that can make the statements inviting in nature. For example, "I am not seeing you help me in the household works, kindly help me with the work."

Choosing Your Battles

If you are willing to start a constructive discussion, you must stick to a single issue at one time. All those couples who are unhappy are most likely to bring in several topics at once. Such practices will not allow the prime issue to enter the boundary, resulting in unsolved problems. Try to solve only one issue at one time. Trying to gulp in a full pizza at once will surely choke you. The same thing applies to relationship conflict discussions. However, a heated conversation can easily turn into a fight where both the partners try to throw mud at each other. It will take the shape of a complaining session eventually. Always remember the more number of complaints you try to raise, the less likely it is going to be to solve any of the problems.

Not Objecting To The Complaints Of Your Partner Automatically

When your partner is criticizing you, it might be hard for you not to turn on the defensive mode. However, defensiveness can never help in solving issues. For example, a couple is arguing where one partner wants the other to get indulged in doing the house chores. The other partner says that he does not have enough time to do so. So, the first partner says that he/she can keep aside some time at the weekend for helping in the house chores to which he/she gets a reply that they would happily do so but have plans with friends at the weekend. This form of 'yes-but' behavior indicates that the first partner's suggestions are not important for the other partner. Another form of defensive behavior, which is destructive in nature, is 'cross-complaining.' It is the act of responding to the complaints of your partner with a complaint of your own. For instance, replying to "You do not help me clean the house" with "You are a neat-maniac."

Getting defensive all the time is not going to help the relationship in any way. It is always important to listen to what your partner wants to say and consider what is being said by them. If you keep turning on the shield and do not pay attention to what is being said, the time is near when the relationship is going to be harmed.

Taking An Alternate Perspective

Along with listening to your partner, you are required to accept the perspective of your partner. You will also need to understand the point of origin of the perspectives. All those who can positively accept their partner's perspective are less likely to get irritated during an issue discussion. Also, you can opt for taking an objective perspective besides the perspective of your partner. As you try to think of a situation from an objective perspective besides your partner's, you can gain more knowledge of any situation. It can also help maintain a stable level of relationship satisfaction as you put in extra effort to understand your partner's side. Understanding each other is all that matters in a relationship.

Not Showing Contempt

Out of all forms of negative things that can you can say and do at the time of a conflict, the worst is contempt. Remarks of contemptuous type are the ones that are used for belittling your partner. It also involves name-calling and sarcasm. It might also involve nonverbal behaviors such as smirking or rolling your eyes. Such types of behaviors are always very disrespectful. It can imply that your partner disgusts you.

Imagine that one of the partners says, "I wish we could go out more." The other partner replies by saying, "Oh, absolutely, all that matters to you is to be seen. You want me to keep paying for all those tiny food portions at some posh restaurant. How much superficial could someone be?" Or one of the partners says they are very much tired for cleaning up the house, to which the other partner replies. "Surely, you are too tired. I have been working the whole day, and now you return home and jump on the couch, staring at your phone. Even a teenager behaves better than you." Contemptuous statements of this kind can easily make it impossible to have a real discussion. Such statements can also ignite the fire of anger in your partner. As a result, no one will opt for a real attempt to solve the actual issue.

Not Getting Overwhelmed With Negativity

It might be tough to respond immediately to your partner's bad behavior with something even worse. However, when you indulge yourself in such an urge, it can make the conflict even worse. Whenever couples tend to engage in negative affect reciprocity, they bring in more heated insults along with contemptuous remarks in the relationship. The more the conflict goes on, the more negativity it escalates. So, what is the measurement f 'too' much negativity? It has been found in research that the magic number of a relationship is a ratio of 5 to 1. In simple terms, you need to maintain a ratio of five good or positive behaviors to each of the negative behavior. Good behaviors can involve anything such as warmth, collaboration, good humor, and many others. As you try to maintain this ratio throughout your relationship, chances are very less of you both getting separated.

Knowing The Time For Time-Out

Whenever you see yourself giving into negative patterns and finding out that you or your partner are not abiding by the tips mentioned above, try taking a time -out from the argument. Try to take a few deep breaths along with your partner for calming your hot tempers. Practicing various ways together for pausing a heated argument can help in saving the relationship from excessive damage.

Chapter 8: Relationship Between Anxiety And Conflicts

When issues start cropping up in your relationship, you might have the feeling that your anxieties are being warranted. You might start feeling that all your worries are coming to be true. Try your best not to get indulged in thoughts of this type. Anxiety generally originates from the unknown. Conflicts tend to arise whenever the expectations or needs are not met, or there are differences in opinions. They might turn out to be healthy if handled in the right way, while anxieties are nothing but harmful. Some of the definite ways in which conflicts can affect anxiety are:

- **Increased heartbeat:** Conflicts result in the release of adrenaline. It can be made worse by anxiety. It might result in a rapid heartbeat, which can slowly escalate to shortness of breath. Conflict, coupled with anxiety, can make these physiological symptoms bad. It takes the structure of a vicious cycle. The best way of combating this is by approaching conflict face to face with calmness. If you can try to avoid being upset, raise your voice, or react in anger, you can easily prevent the trigger of an adrenaline rush. It can successfully suppress the anxiety feelings.

- **Nervous movement or energy:** Again, adrenaline rush comes into play. You will feel your body suddenly getting filled with excessive energy that needs to be used somehow. As at the time of an argument, you are most likely not to fight or run, the energy gets transformed into pacing, hand wringing, toe-tapping, along with certain other nervous movements. All these might turn out to be very disturbing for your partner and also yourself when you are in the mid-way of a conflict. Indeed, the fault is not yours. But the knowledge of the same will not make it fade away. All you can do is to face the situation with a calm mind for preventing the adrenaline rush.

Anxiety And Panic Attacks

Anxiety can effectively lead to panic and anxiety attacks, which is nothing new. But you need to remember that while conflicts occur, it is for your good that you keep calm if you have problems with panic and anxiety. Such situations can easily trigger an attack, which can make everything go worse. Anxiety and panic attacks are generally characterized by:

- Sweating
- Difficulty breathing
- Difficulty concentrating
- Feeling of unknown doom
- Racing thoughts

Although there is nothing new to say, these symptoms are not funny. So, you need to be mindful before getting into an argument that if you fail to be level headed, you might face an attack.

__Being Defensive__

Nothing can be more destructive to the constructive resolution of conflicts than the habit of defensiveness. Anxiety can effectively block out the rational portion of your mind that plays the part of thinking about a situation with logic. When this logic is not present, you might face a tough time in focusing on what is being said by your partner. You are most likely to shift your focus from listening to lashing out. You will turn out the defensive shield, even in situations when your partner is not attacking you. You should definitely defend your position when you are being treated unjustly. However, if your partner is willing to opt for a peaceful resolution of the issues, the best action is to match up with their intentions. You will need to drop your defensive shield for the betterment of the relationship. But when you are having anxious thoughts, doing all these is not going to be easy.

Shut Down

In place of just turning on your defensive mode, you might choose to shut down completely. Your anxious mind might find it tough to process all those things that are happening. The lack of energy during the situation can lead to a complete shutdown. As such a thing happens, you will not be able to concentrate or focus. You will not be able to call out rationality or logic for working through the conflict. Also, you will not be able to comprehend what is being said by your partner. You will be feeling empty and heavy on the inside, feeling like a battery that has drained suddenly. The best thing that can be done on your side in such a situation is to relax and mend. Conflicts will be in place unless you can take back the control over your mind and activate rationality.

How To Successfully Overcome A Bad Relationship Dispute?

When you face a conflict in your healthy and growing relationship, try to think about how you can talk or express your feelings regarding this conflict. The primary aim is to establish a good communication model. Good communication is where every individual can check the stock and get an idea about the other person's attitude. The conflict resolution will seem a lot easier to manage when it is not escalated with unnecessary things such as angry tones. For effective communication during conflicts, you will need to follow three simple rules:

- Keep your calm and do not raise your voice.
- Let your partner talk. Let them develop the state of the argument, as communication not only includes talking but listening also.
- Try to reach a middle ground; however, do not opt for compromises that can negatively affect the coming days.

A couple who has the habit of arguing and respects all these rules can easily reach a resolution.

Required Actions For Overcoming Conflicts Between Partners

Relationships are not meant to be easy. You will keep learning when you are in a healthy relationship. Is it even possible to not repeat the mistakes and stabilize the base of your romantic relationship? Is it possible to manage the relationship conflicts without you being hurt? Try to follow all these recommendations for rebuilding the love in your struggling relationship.

- After you are well aware of the reasons behind the relationship tensions that tend to shake the relationship base, you can focus on moving to a more 'direct' phase of harmony. Yes, the first phase might turn out to be very psychological, as you will need to communicate with the other person. However, it is necessary if you want to bring back your relationship on its track.
- It is important to use more thoughtful and technical actions to find your partner's heart. It is also needed to overcome the relationship crisis.
- The actions that you decide upon to use needs to correspond with various issues. Otherwise, your actions will not have any kind of effect on the situation. It can even aggravate the issues. Do not just opt for resolution for the sake of being done with it; opt for resolution for making the situations better.
- Do not keep assigning blame to the other side. A relationship is not a one-man game. It is all about team effort. Both the partners are required to be in the relationship fully. If one of the partners keeps on giving effort while the other just sits idle, it will be better for the relationship to not even exist.

- If you or your partner is not feeling satisfied or fulfilled in your relationship, you are required to spend more time together. It will help you both to understand the problems in a better way. You will also come to know what you both want and need from the relationship.

Every relationship in this world is bound to go through conflicts at some point or the other. All that is important for you to know is that disagreements are not always a bad thing. It is how individuals in relationships try to express their varying views on a topic or situation.

Compromising As A Common Solution

The use of compromise in relationships is very common for resolving disputes and disagreements in the mediation and negotiation process. While it can lead to the production of an agreement, compromise is not powerful enough for resolving conflicts all the time. It cannot work specifically in situations when there are some underlying organizational or interpersonal conflicts. The prime reason for this is that compromise is a settled resolution to an issue. It is not at all the ultimate solution which is sought by either partner. It can effectively generate a material or a functional solution. But it cannot resolve behavioral or emotional issues that are coupled with disagreements. As the end result, either one of the partners or both will continue to carry forward certain ill feelings or dissatisfaction that might come to the surface once again if the same nature of issue arises.

Compromise is being defined as a win/lose agreement where both the partners tend to get something of what they wish for. But it is not possible to attain everything that they want. The majority of the tensions or issues crop up with a collaborative or competitive strategy. The outcome that is best possible in such a situation is the ultimate goal of both partners. But various other important factors come in the equation such as financial cost, time requirement, practical matters, and use of power. The ultimate realization that the desired outcomes might turn out to be unachievable can force the partners to opt for a process of negotiation. It involves the concept of give and take for reaching a mutual agreement of compromised nature.

Agreeing To Disagree

Using compromise for settling a dispute or conflict needs both the partners involved to be aware that the result might be less than what they hoped for. The ultimate decision might be the one that is acceptable, however, not optimal. You may feel resistance or reluctance to use compromise to resolve conflicts when you think the result will be a loss. When the primary focus is on things that are achieved, instead of things that have been given up, chances of acceptance and satisfaction of both partners is high. Compromise will turn out to be a successful venture if both partners have a choice of tangible outcomes. The outcomes are required to be open for consideration so that the final decision is something that always remains within a common box for both partners.

There might be a requirement to 'agree to disagree' at some point in cases when the issues seem incurable and the realization that they will be unable to agree completely sets in. Agreeing to disagree is essential when the disagreement is over principles or values rather than methods or facts. When both partners can learn to listen to each other and respectfully understand the other person's point, accepting the disagreements will seem a lot easier. A mutual form of acceptance regarding the differences can improve the likelihood of a proper resolution to any issue or dispute.

Compromise can turn out to be a perfect and effective method for resolving differences and conflicts. However, it might not be the right choice all the time. Opting for compromise, even when other modes of conflict seem more appropriate, can lead to an outcome that is of no use for the current situation. You will need to make sure that significant requirements or vital issues are not lost during the process of compromise. Sometimes you might need to opt for other creative solutions. All forms of disagreements and differences are not needed to be negotiated.

When Is Compromise Regarded As An Appropriate Move?

Using the card of compromise to resolve issues or disputes is regarded as appropriate in the listed situations:

- When the prime differences have been effectively identified, and there is a requirement to move forward.
- When the relationship's general health will benefit from both partners, sacrificing some of their needs or demands.
- When it does not feel like real to satisfy both partners who are involved in the issue.
- When there is a need for quick resolution, even if the resolution is temporary.
- When the demands or needs of both partners have equal merit and importance.

Resolving Disputes With The Help Of Compromise

When one partner comes with a thinking preference while the other comes with feeling orientation for decision making, the chances are high that there will be a disagreement in using compromise for resolving a conflict. The partner with thinking preference will try to use facts and logic for proving their points with the motive of proving the other person wrong. The partner who is a 'feeler' might get driven by their emotional values and energy that will make them defensive. They will try their best to be on their point instead of opting for compromise. In such a case, both partners can opt for a mediator. In simple terms, both partners will demonstrate their points to a third person who will try to bring fairness and understanding in the conflict.

When both partners are the 'feeler' type, the option of compromise might not be brought in the picture by either partner. They might feel more inclined to invest in collaboration to meet the demands of both sides. However, this option might not work out sometimes. When both partners are 'feeler,' they must be subjective and objective in their examination of the circumstances and possible outcomes. When you and your partner decide to compromise, make sure each of you gives up on something of equal importance or value. This way, you can balance both sides of the negotiation.

Chapter 9: Strategies For Improving Existing Relationships

When you decide to strengthen a relationship, try to give your best for improving the connection. If you have already found the individual with whom you would like to spend the rest of your life and want to start the relationship on the right foot, there are certain points that you will need to remember.

- **Have common values and visions:** If one of you keeps spending all the time while the other keeps saving money, if one of you keeps maintaining a proper diet while the other keeps having junk foods, if one of you is on one side of the political spectrum while the other is on either side, etc., the chances are high that fights will keep taking place. Such differences will lead to frequent conflicts. For lasting the relationship, you will need to prepare a set of commonalities for which both of you can come together. Try to have a common vision that will help you and your partner project the relationship into a shining future. Doing this will help in sharing dreams and will also establish a good understanding between partners.

- **Please each other and try to give recognition:** The most common thing that tends to destroy the majority of the relationships is when partners take each other for granted. When you stop yourself from putting in efforts into the relationship, you take the relationship for granted. For example, when you do not try to nurture your relationship, when you keep criticizing now and then, when you do not pay attention to the struggles of your partner, and when you have the belief that your partner will love you without even doing anything for the relationship. It is not the way how relationships work out. For both partners in a healthy relationship to feel appreciated and loved, both partners need to recognize each other. You are required to show gratitude to your partner and vice versa. This type of attitude can help nurture collaboration, encourage a steady connection, and help the partners appreciate each other. No matter what happens in the relationship, never take your partner and the relationship for granted.

- **Be proud of your partner:** Is it possible to live happily in a relationship if you cannot even admire your partner? The answer is no. There is no need for your romantic partner to win a Nobel Prize or a trophy for being praised by the person whom they love, which is you. If you cannot even appreciate at least a single trait of your partner, no matter if it is beauty, intelligence, courage, determination, or humor, you do not appreciate your partner's existence in your life. Human beings tend to gravitate towards all those who express acceptance, love, and fulfillment towards them. Give your best efforts to make your romantic partner feel accepted and loved all the time. Just appreciate him/her in the relationship, and you will be able to maintain the spark in your relationship.
- **Try having realistic expectations:** Some women are always searching for an impossible Prince Charming. They tend to believe that romantic relationships will always look like a fairy tale. Talking about men, they might get influenced by the standards that are being set by the media. No matter what sort of unfounded expectations you keep inside yourself, if they tend to be unrealistic, they are most likely to generate

disappointment in your relationship. It is always better to have modest and realistic expectations regarding your relationship. Always remember, a relationship is not an easy game. You will need to fight various obstacles for giving it a proper shape. So, instead of just setting up unrealistic expectations, try to shift your focus on the betterment of the relationship. It will be better for you and your partner too.

When you feel happy with all that you have got, you are bound to feel satisfied. If you always try to look for someone better for replacing your partner, without paying attention to the genuine qualities, you will harm the relationship in all possible means. Doing so will make you feel lost in your illusion that can be found in your imagination only.

- **Provide affection daily:** It has been found that long-lasting relationships are the ones in which the partners have been capable of replacing passion and love gradually with attachment. The majority of the people are not even aware of it, but the neurotransmitters and hormones determine most of our behaviors. Affection, tenderness, and cuddling help in oxytocin production, which is the hormone responsible for attachment. If you are willing to feed in your partner's well-being, never forget to show the power of affection.

- **Do not allow the sexual flame to blow out:** The initial phases of a relationship are always filled with passion and affection. With passing time, the frequency of making love to your partner gets reduced gradually. All of this can be the result of various reasons, for which you cannot blame each other. If this continues, sexual desire will slowly get extinguished. You will find it tough to reignite the spark, no matter how much you try. Sexual desire plays an important role in the well-being of a relationship. The real key to this problem is to give enough time for intimacy in the relationship. Regardless of how busy you are throughout the day, keep showing small gestures that can help keep the spark alive. For example, text your partner to be ready before you reach home, plan a romantic candlelight dinner, text your partner that you love them, appreciate your partner's body, and many others. It all depends on the small gestures that can make a relationship successful.

Exercise daily, eat well, and stay healthy for keeping the flame ignited despite the passing time. The taste of the partners is another thing that also comes into play. It can easily fit into a more generalized vision that can also benefit your health and personal development.

- **Being open about improving yourself:** If both partners keep living in a constant state of self-denial and pride, the relationship is preparing for doom. Being in a healthy relationship means improving yourself every day, opting for compromises, understanding the mistakes and shortcomings, and giving your best for correcting them. People who have the habit of being proud of themselves all the time generally avoid this subject intentionally. They try to move their focus from all the faults and mistakes. If you have such a habit, your partner will find it difficult to be in a relationship. You will need to learn to improve yourself daily. As you keep being proud of yourself, you will gradually shift your attention from your partner towards you. If you are willing to develop a healthy relationship, acknowledge your mistakes, and you can see your relationship reaching new heights.

- **Staying faithful:** Being faithful indicates going out of the boundary of egotism. Being egoistic will make you prioritize your pleasures while keeping aside the needs and interests of your partner. If you think that you truly love a person, deceiving that person will be the last thought on your mind. Love is the richest experience of our lives that needs to be lived with hardships and happiness. Why undermine the value of love with unfaithfulness and lies? In simple terms, romantic relationships are dynamic, just like life. For enriching such relationships, you will need to first acknowledge that your point of view is not the ultimate point of view.

Empathy, respect, and communication can result in a more satisfying relationship without constantly being right. No one can avoid conflicts in healthy relationships. Two different individuals who bring in varying life experiences to the big table are bound to have disagreements. However, when you always try to achieve the goals you want to, without paying attention to what the other partner needs, you tend to get engaged in certain behaviors that will only lead to a breakup. It might feel like a real challenge to bring various motivations together via common values. But you also have got a large tool for meeting this challenge: communication.

For sharing the rest of your life with an individual, basic wisdom needs you to make certain sacrifices. When you opt for not communicating with your partner, even if your goal is to keep away conflicts at any cost, you will end up achieving disastrous results.

It does not matter if you are with your partner for a long or short time. Strong connections are bound to form when you learn to accept your responsibility to make an effort and understand your partner's point of view.

Tips For Improving The Bond

Indeed, each relationship is unique, but no relationship is exquisite. By following these tips for improving your relationship bond, you will not only guarantee a great connection with your partner but will also make sure that you want to work for resolving the conflicts.

Start By Asking Your Partner Something New

Communication is always regarded as the measurement of togetherness in all forms of relationships. It is a pleasant thing to ask your partner how their day went. But it might result to be exhausting if you keep asking them the same question every day. Ensure that you do not turn your relationship communication into something redundant or boring. It is a joint game for keeping yourself engaged in the relationship with varying dialogues that are meaningful and engaging at the same time.

Fix A Month To Month Plan For Night Out

Regardless of your busy schedule, make sure that you plan a special night where the two of you will get some time to spend together. Try to be devoted and consistent with it after you agree on a date with your romantic partner. If you are willing to add some spice to your relationship or try out something new apart from Netflix, leaving the house's boundary is a more promising act. More number of memories can be created in the world out of our couch. Spend time together and devote time to make new memories. Memories can help n reigniting the spark of a relationship when there is nothing new to be done. You can fix a particular date every month when you and your partner will go on a long drive, movie night, candlelight dinner, explore new places, and many others. The aim is to spend the maximum amount of time with each other. Whenever you find the spark of your relationship fading away, plan something new.

Expressing Appreciation

The consolation offered by a relationship is the prime reason we will generally not pay attention to all those things that our partner does. We will treat their affection demonstration as compulsory. In simple terms, your partner is not bound to get your favorite juice or fill your gas tank. They think of doing so only because they love you. When you learn to recognize and appreciate your partner's gestures towards you, you will be able to strengthen the base of the relationship. You will be able to make your partner feel inspired to be attentive. It takes nothing to appreciate the small gestures made by your partner. Appreciation is something that can easily determine the future of a relationship.

Lack of appreciation from your side will make your partner reduce their effort to dedicate to the relationship. It will ultimately lead to the drowning of the relationship. No matter what your partner does for you or the relationship, just appreciate their effort. Also, make sure that you get back the same from your partner as you try to do something for them and the relationship. A relationship is both a side game.

Changing The Timetable

Everyone in this world is autonomous, and it will be completely wrong to expect someone to cease the flow of their life for someone else. Indeed, you have various other responsibilities outside the boundary of your relationship. But it can always help if you keep a check on your schedule and see if there are any kinds of conflicts that are stopping you from spending time with your partner. Maybe you can ask your partner to visit the gym early so that you can both make it to the late-night movie show, or you can simply wake up early for finishing all your tasks and then dedicate the rest of the time for helping your partner. There is no need to completely forfeit your personal life for fulfilling your partner's life.

However, your capability to bargain with your life for taking out some time is enough to satisfy your partner. Whenever you get the chance to alter your schedule for dedicating that time to your partner, just do it. But remember not to give up on your own life. You can also involve your partner within your schedule for sharing some together time.

Demonstrating Your Love

Besides appreciating your partner, you must learn how to explain your extent of love to your partner. You can express your part of love for your partner with various simple gestures, such as holding hands while walking on the road, staring at your partner while sipping on your coffee at a café, and many others. Such gestures will not only depict your love for your partner. They can also help in indicating that you are appreciative and proud of having your partner. There is no need to do something grand all the time to express your love. Simple gestures can do the task easily. Sometimes even a smile at your partner while you both stand at two different corners in a party is enough for demonstrating your love.

"I love you," a small phrase that everyone loves to hear from their partner's mouth. These three little words come with the capability of making your partner feel special and loved. It can help in attracting your partner closer to you as a real bond. Saying those three little words every day to your partner, as you wake up in the morning, or when your partner is cooking in the kitchen, can help in making the bond stronger. However, make sure that you say them honestly, from your heart, and not as a mere habit. Expressing your love for your partner is not required to be elaborate. All that it needs is to be sincere. You can show your love for your partner by kissing them, giving surprise gifts, or hugging each other. It is the smallest things that build a relationship, and not something grand all the time.

Getting Familiar With The Behavior Of Your Partner

Does your partner like to be left alone whenever they feel disturbed? How does your partner react in certain situations? All these inquiries about your partner are basic. The responses to all these can help you comprehend your partner's behavior. You can also prevent yourself from getting offended by your partner suddenly. How your partner sees the world is not at all the same way as you do. So, how your partner reacts to different situations will also be different from yours. Just learn about their behavioral traits. If your partner loves to spend some alone time whenever they feel annoyed, prevent yourself from pestering your partner. The aim is to make yourself aware of all the behavioral traits of your partner. It will help in preventing conflicts and bring in harmony. Getting used to your partner's behaviors will also make your partner feel that you understand their traits and values.

Learning When To Say Sorry

You will need to understand that being correct is not of the same significance as being sympathetic. Clashes are bound to occur in relationships, but there are certain arguments required to be won. I am trying to explain that you are required to know what is worth fighting for and when you are required to accept the mistake. It is always a better option to apologize and say sorry than turning a tiny argument into a serious crisis that might break the relationship. Whenever you make any mistake, own up to it, and apologize for the same. Apologizing won't hurt your image. It will depict that you are a person who is brave enough to own their mistakes. There is nothing shameful in saying sorry to the person you love. Do not turn on your defensive shield and take up all the blame for your mistakes.

Going To Bed Together

Most couples do not opt for ending the day together. Often, one of the partners stays awake lately in a separate room watching TV or browsing the internet, while the other sleeps in bed. It has been found that couples who have different sleeping schedules and are not habituated with going to bed together tend to grow detached from each other. It can easily result in feelings of loneliness in the relationship. It can directly make couples drift apart from each other. The time that you get in bed is the time that you get to spend with each other through touch. Your body will release oxytocin, known as the love hormone, which will make you get close to your partner. It is the prime time when the majority of the couples try to get intimate physically. Not only physical intimacy, but you also get the chance to share your experiences throughout the day with your partner. Cuddling during bedtime has shown some seriously positive effects on relationship bonding. So, if you have some kind of work to finish before going to bed, ask your partner to stay awake for some time.

Being Honest All The Time

When you get into a relationship, you dedicate yourself to your partner, and vice versa. One of the tips for making your bond stronger is to always be honest with your partner. When you try to be honest with your mate, you can make your partner feel that they can trust you. Being honest does not always mean telling the truth. It also involves the act of honoring your romantic partner with deed and words. Honesty in relationships also comes with various other benefits. For instance, you cannot read the mind of your partner. When you practice being honest with each other, you can open up a new window of healthy communication. You can effortlessly express all your feelings and fix any existing problems with ease.

If you want to say something to your partner, say it directly. Do not opt for indirect means for conveying your feelings or thoughts. For example, if you do not like your partner's certain behavior, just speak up about the same directly. Direct conversations can help in resolving conflicts much easier than anything else. The aim is to be transparent with each other.

Get Rid Of The Past

As being a culprit for several potential conflicts and other underlying issues for the future ones, all those things that happen in the past will not stay there. It will be very difficult for you to move ahead in a healthy relationship if you keep thinking about an issue from the past. Doing so will prevent you from making any future gestures. Suppose you see yourself continuously dwelling in the past. In that case, it is a definite sign of taking one step back and just consider 'why.' Do you have the nature of being less forgiving, or did something happen in the past that is not allowing you to forgive? As you focus all your attention on the reason for this sort of recurring feeling, you will be able to gain more clarity regarding the situation. You will get a clear picture of yourself and what do you need from the relationship with your partner.

Practical Exercises And Lessons

A healthy relationship can always make your life feel a lot better. Stop, and think for a moment, all the suffering, stress that you always experience whenever you have a conflict in your relationship. So, it can be said that your life gets improved in all possible means when you opt for harmony in your romantic relationship. This exercise is a kind of self-diagnosis that can help you gain more knowledge about the things that need to be improved for bringing in harmony. Try to opt for the exercise with your partner. Use the process of evaluation for discussing the various to improve. Provide a percentage between 0 – 100% besides each of the below-mentioned aspects, where 0% is little or never, and 100% is a lot or always.

Relational dimensions concerning you as a couple:

- Your ability to listen to each other:
- Your ability to speak and participate in exchanges:
- Your ability to be empathetic (putting yourself in your partner's shoes and understanding their aspect):
- You ability to express love, gratitude, etc.:
- Your ability to support one another at the time of difficulties:
- Your ability to approach your partner regarding the improvement of your relationship:

After you have successfully provided percentage for all, try to concentrate on how you can improve those aspects with the lowest score.

Questions For Identifying The Weaknesses And Strengths Of The Relationship

As you answer all the below mentioned questions, you will be able to be aware of the gaps in your relationship that need to be filled together along with the positive aspects for which gratitude can be maintained.

- What are the things that you like the most in your relationship?
- What is your extent of affection and intimacy as a couple?
- What are those things that you feel unsatisfied with? What are the things that you are missing in the relationship?
- Is the degree of intimacy and affection enough to satisfy you?

After you are done with answering all these questions, let's look at some more useful strategies that can help nurture all your desires in the relationship. It can also help to make your relationship last forever. You might think that is it even possible to achieve so? The answer is yes, you can. All that it involves is a bit of hard work and dedication. Indeed, it won't be feeling like magic all the time. However, you can easily develop new skills for being happy together in your relationship. Always remember, you are in this together. So, whatever new things you try for the relationship, it needs to be mutual.

- **Try to be in love with yourself:** You will never be happy in your relationship if you cannot be happy with yourself. Love is meant to be offered first to yourself and then to others. Learn to be happy as the person you are. Try to know more about yourself and make every effort to accept yourself. It is quite easy to set up a beautiful intimacy with your internal world. Feel strong, confident, and be proud of who you are. It might seem like a challenger, but it is necessary at the same time. All you need to do is to care for the presence of yourself. The more richness you can bring in your life and you are dipped in the energy of compassion for yourself, the more you will be able to love others. You can truly love your romantic partner when you love yourself in the first place.

It can be said that the love you have in store to offer is directly proportional to the amount of love you have in store for yourself. When there is an absence of this movement related to tenderness and gratitude for yourself, you will risk searching for someone who can fill the void or the gaps that you think you have. Two complete people coming together can always make a better and healthy relationship than two people looking for filling their voids.

- **Proper investment in the relationship:** A committed form of love is a love where you always invest your all in the relationship. You can think of your romantic relationship as a plant. If you want the plant to be healthy and beautiful, you will need to take proper care of the same. The same thing goes for our relationships. You will need to maintain its health for keeping it alive. You will need to invest your time and attention to help it grow and sustain. The majority of the time, couples tend to end their relationship only because they failed to take care of the bonding properly. It is not the love that tends to fail; it is the effort. It is nothing but an evident problem of negligence. Just like a plant, a relationship that is not maintained properly fades, becomes weak, and will die eventually.

For succeeding in a relationship, you and your partner need to dedicate energy and time into the relationship. We, as human beings, can take our partner for granted very easily. We get lost in our daily schedules and life business. Our schedules are so much filled with other stuff that there is no space available for sharing with our relationship. It will eventually create emotional famine and result in depletion of the connection. There are some important pointers that can be used for nourishing your relationship:

1. Take at least half an hour to discuss your mood and day with your partner every day.
2. Dedicate time for working on projects together.
3. Try to do special activities together at least once a month.
4. Express your affection, gratitude, and commitment towards your partner daily.
5. Take care of one another with small delicacies, touches, and surprises.

- **Love is more of a commitment than a feeling:** Love in a sustainable and healthy relationship is much more than sparks in your eyes and butterflies in the stomach. The majority of us possess a rustic vision of romantic love. We tend to think that love, at first sight, is a guarantee of a forever lasting relationship. The passion is required to be maintained all along, at any cost. Otherwise, we will just conclude that the love has gone and the separation is inevitable. In actual, genuine love is not the result of hormones gone crazy or chemical reactions in the brain. It results from a dedicated effort of appreciating one another even when you feel the 'spark' is missing. True love is capable of passing from the elevated feelings in the start to a stable and solid companionship in ordinary, daily life. Investing in a nurturing and happy relationship needs effort, perseverance, and determination.

It is necessary to keep in mind that love is meant to meet one of the basic needs: to feel emotionally safe. So, when love results from mutual commitment, it tends to be very safe. This form of security will allow you and your romantic partner to stand hand in hand all across the life trails. You will come to understand that you have someone by your side to lean on when your life does not feel right.

- **Genuine communication:** Effective communication is the prime key to the success of a healthy love life. The more you and your partner can create emotional weather of security and trust between you two; the more self-revelation will be possible. However, it is, among all other things, the extent of exchanges that helps in binding you together. It helps in encouraging intimacy. You can discuss the weather and the rain with your friends and colleagues. But, try to aim for something more meaningful with your romantic partner. This form of sharing, coupled with depth and authenticity, can help bring two individuals closer by permitting them to feel solidarity with one another and be in sync. This type of deep connection is one of the primary goals of a healthy relationship. The aim is to feel connected to one another emotionally, which you can enjoy more than other things.

There are some strategies that you can opt for to promote good communication.

1. Take full responsibility for the course of your life.
2. Open up about your emotions and express clearly what you need. Do not leave your partner with the guessing game.
3. Avoid as much as you can to accuse your partner.
4. Learn to listen to your partner. Do not opt for a response all the time. Just listen sometimes.
5. Always express compassion and empathy for all the things that your partner tells.
6. Try to avoid the subjects of taboo. They can readily poison your relationship.

- **Try to change yourself rather than changing your partner:** There is no greater mirror that can show you all your flaws than your relationship. While your partner can help bring out the best in you, they can also indirectly make you see your worst. This thing goes both ways: we do not seem to recognize all our flaws until another individual sees them. It might be difficult to submit yourself to the vulnerability that tends to come while being in a mutual relationship and getting to know that you are not perfect. At times, we try to use up this vulnerability against our partner, changing all those things that we do not like. We shift our focus from all those things that we can change about us. Our pride stays side by side with our ego while comfortably indulging in blindness and denial.

Indeed, willing to bring about some changes in someone else is an ineffective wish. You have power only over yourself. It depends on you, whether you are prone to heal and transform the flaws in yourself. Relationships can be regarded as a great opportunity to heal the wounds that you possess, even when it is very scary to dwell where it aches. What if you shift your focus to yourself instead of blaming your partner? What if you can recognize that you can opt for something good for the relationship's health by concentrating on your inner self? You will be able to change the definition of your relationship. You can see your bond in new colors. Just try it once. You will feel amazed after seeing the results.

- **Admiring your partner:** Always believe in the potential of your partner. Support them as they work on implementing all their dreams. No matter if it is five or thirty years that you walk hand in hand, the goal will still be the same- to be always there for one another. Try to maintain a positive perspective of who your romantic partner is. Try to have faith in who they are trying to be. This form of movement involving profound complicity will allow you both to support each other in your quest for meaningful existence and happiness. I know that the challenge is really great. You will start seeing only those things that tend to get on the nerves, too easily. However, do not lose your focus from the complete picture.

Love is a form of commitment that needs plenty of maturity, investment, and will. You will need to change your focus from criticizing your partner and their activities. Instead of criticizing, try to acknowledge the accomplishments of your partner regularly. Opt for seeing the glass as half full and not as half empty. The aim is to appreciate your partner, no matter what they do or achieve. Just like a 'perfect' human, a 'perfect' partner also can never be found. In fact, it does not even exist. The life of being a couple is a ceaseless dance of adjustments, letting go, and compromise. Happiness can be achieved as we try to prepare a bouquet only with those flowers that we possess.

- **Choosing the arguments wisely:** Let us be realistic; it is almost inevitable in a relationship that is intimate, which tends to affect all the life spheres; there will be issues over the ways of doing and seeing things. Life with someone else tends to aggravate all the differences. It is idealistic to look for harmony and proper agreement in every area of life. There will be struggles, but all of them are not bad. So, how can you argue in a way that is healthy?
    1. Keep in mind that the other person is whom you love. He/she is not your enemy.

2. Always try to work as one team and not as two different competitors.
3. Make best efforts for avoiding sterile dynamics: "Who is right, and who is wrong?"
4. Do not just opt for a war but search for "win-win" solutions.
5. Try to defuse the conflicts much early before they can escalate.
6. Your love life is a duet dance, not a war.
7. Try not to use words that tend to destroy: hatred, revenge, punishment.
8. View the differences as enrichments and not as obstacles.
9. Try to nourish your bond of intimate attachment, even at times of conflicts.
10. Address your conflicts gently and calmly. It helps in improving the chances of positive solutions.

You need to be judgmental enough while bringing up any argument. If the argument isn't going to help the state of your relationship in any way, it will be better not to start such arguments. Try to discuss all those issues that you think need to be resolved while being in a relationship. The same goes for your romantic companion as well.

- **Love is human:** Why are there so many questions when it comes to love? Why is love always so tough? What are the things that make physical intimacy with your romantic partner so demanding? There are multiple factors that can explain the high repetition of difficulties whenever it comes to success in a healthy relationship. One of the important things that need to be highlighted: the dilemma between our human side and our animal side. Although, as being humans, we always claim that we are very superior and advanced than other creations on this planet. But we should also not forget our animal side that is never too far away. The brain part, the hypothalamus, which we often call refer to as the reptilian brain, is being programmed in a way so that we can survive. Our survival solely depends on the protections against odds and dangers. In your romantic relationship, you might sometime think of your partner as the danger.

  In such a situation, your mechanism of survival will call for the guarding of your territory. There is nothing doubtful that we are programmed biologically to respond to our needs and react negatively to all those things that might seem a threat to our lives. Fortunately, human beings have also been provided with emotional and rational intelligence. At the bottom of your humanity, you are a caring, loving, and fundamentally good creature. Don't you think it is the ultimate human evolution that needs to be loved?

It depends on you which of the two sides you want to prioritize. Which one do you think will win? For walking towards the best version of yourself, you will need to be open to the presence and awareness of all your inner tensions or issues. For loving your partner truly, you will first need to undertake the task of healing your wounds from past love and all your scars of defense. This form of transformation will make it possible for you to acquire a great sense of maturity, both psychologically and emotionally. This form of maturity is certainly essential for a sustainable and healthy love life. Always opt for the human side, and put love in the first place.

- **Power is worth dividing:** The prime issues that come in the life of partners are from power. We all want it. We want to hold it. We aspire for it. We all demand to be heard, seen, recognized, and to make a steady place in the ever-changing world. We tend to fight for claiming our space. In a relationship, you and your partner belong to the same team. Both of your share and exist in the same territory. It can create an inevitable struggle for power if you fail to see the partnership as an effective joint effort. It might, in some of the cases, be balanced and healthy. However, in some relationships, the power struggle tends to turn destructive and toxic. The partners who belong to the same team turn into enemies. They start playing against one another. The duet becomes a duel. For example, when a couple keeps quarreling about something very simple, such as how to arrange the clothes in the wardrobe, the problem is not with the clothes, but the power.

The proper distribution of power can be found in various dimensions of our daily lives. The right division of tasks is a prime issue that is sensitive as well. It is often the first ground of tensions and conflicts between couples. Moreover, it has been found that couples who have the habit of a division of labor last longer in love. It is a simple question of equity and justice.

- **Avoiding the worst things that you can do:** It is important to conclude this section with all those things that you will need to avoid at any cost in a healthy relationship. Do not accuse, criticize, or humiliate your romantic partner when you both are fighting. It will only add fuel to the conflict fire and will act as inauguration music of war. If you are willing to play this game, there will only be losers. There is an effective way of managing all your tensions without pushing yourself towards devastation and falling prey to the lowest instincts. Start by watching out for violent words. Such words can easily leave back marks that cannot be removed. It will take you some seconds to say them. But it will take months or even years to heal your partner's wounds that you have caused with your words.

  It is not a great idea to escape issues by choosing to sulk or being silent. These types of withdrawal attitudes will only be aggravating the whole situation. They will damage instead of improving your connection. A classic scenario in all the unhealthy relationship dynamics often looks like: one of the partners will express his/her discontent, and the other partner will stop listening and just withdraw into their caves. The more one of the partners tends to withdraw, the more amount of frustration it will accumulate. The more one of the partners manifests their distress, the more the other partner will isolate him/her. It will ultimately result in a blow-up. It will end taking the structure of a toxic spiral that keeps going on and on. The partners will be transformed into two different solitudes that will suffer. When this spiral takes the chronic form, it will mark the starting of the end.

We all are fundamental beings of love and relationships. We have been made to love and to be loved. Two partners' lives are always regarded as a privilege as they can experience a nourishing and secure intimacy. Being attuned to each other will always help in making the relationship happier. You will be able to enjoy better psychological as well as physical health. So, it is worthwhile to start believing in the same and investing in a healthy relationship.

Chapter 10: Cultivating Healthy And Brand New Relationships

Love comes with its pitfalls. What seems at the beginning, like life on a fluffy cloud, will take no time in changing to a life of struggle and conflict. Love is not only about the feeling of having sparks and butterflies in your stomach. Maintaining genuine love needs hard work. But in the end, it gets paid well with satisfaction and happiness. The tips that you will find in this chapter will help you in having a relationship that can elegantly bypass all the typical friction points. In this chapter, you will learn several ways to recognize and take care or true love. Love can change the behaviors and attitudes of human beings. It is exciting, intoxicating, and also scary at times. Love is not always a feeling of delusion and lust. It is something more in all possible senses of feeling.

Allowing Vulnerability

One of the definite signs of falling in love is the moment when you feel vulnerable suddenly. This form of vulnerability can be seen easily in your longings, fears, and feelings. As you start falling in love, your door of heart will open in front of your partner. You will start entrusting your heart to your romantic partner. You will begin to showcase yourself in front of them, as you tend to do with only those close to you. You might feel a bit worried about being vulnerable, specifically if you had bad experiences in your past relationships. When you are vulnerable and open, all those issues that were suppressed otherwise by you might come under your consciousness in a new relationship. So, there might be an underlying fear that will try to scare you. But do not submit to your fears. In a new relationship, everything is new. As you keep judging them, depending on your previous experiences, it will not be fair to them and also to you.

Selflessness

Another definite sign of falling in love is selflessness. It happens when both the partners put both of their needs in priority while subordinating their self needs. You will tend to everything that you have in power to make sure that your partner is happy. This, in turn, provide your partner with a feeling of being cared for. It will make you feel happy as you have successfully acknowledged your partner's needs and fulfilled them.

Actual Beauty Comes From Inside

A very definite sign of being in love is the capability of seeing the inner beauty of your partner. During the initial days of a relationship, most of the attention is provided to outer beauty. As time goes by, as your love feelings start to blossom, you will start paying attention to your partner's actual personality. You will learn to see their true internal beauty. With this thought, the saying 'love can make you go blind' is confirmed.

One-sided relationships can never help you. Even when you feel that living without your partner is not possible for you, and you keep them loving without any measure, unless both of you are on the same page, the relationship is aimless.

How To Cultivate A Meaningful Relationship In The Early Stages?

Let us learn some ways of cultivating healthy and meaningful relationships in the initial stages.

- **Being clear about your needs:** As you meet your partner for the first time, both of you need to examine what you need from a relationship truly. Try to be as clear as you can regarding all that you want. This way, you can be on the same page with your partner from the start. The concept of this might seem alarming, but always learn to expect unexpected things. Your partner might also disclose similar needs or wants.

- **Have open communication:** If you feel troubled with something, try not to hold the same inside you. If you just keep it inside, it can lead to a paranoid fear. Try to address the problems and have caring, quite discussions for seeing your partner's point of view. It is important for discussing together even minute issues so that they do not turn into something big. It does not depend on being right or wrong; it is all about working together as a couple. As you address any issue with joint effort, finding resolutions will seem a lot easier. Just communicate what you are feeling with your partner.

- **Discussing your wants and dreams:** Is your dream to build a small house on your own and live away from the city? Want to take a holiday of one year to travel every corner of the planet? Do you want to write a book? Always share all your dreams with your romantic partner. Try to discover whether all your objectives can complement the objectives of your partner's. Try to find out if you both have common interests. It will turn out to be more fun when you start finding out the dreams of a person rather than discussing their general hobbies.

- **Accepting the minute aspects of yourself:** If you cannot accept who you are, how can you expect someone else to accept you? We all have some specific aspects of ourselves that we do not like or the ones that we would like to change if possible. However, they are not important. The sooner you will be able to take a look at yourself and try to be happy with all those things that you see, the better you can do with your love and life.

- **Talking about major things:** Discuss everything, from getting married to building your own home, from family travels to funds and children. Do not just wait for all these to happen. Try getting a head start and discuss the expectations of both of you from the early stages. Most couples try to avoid discussions of this sort as they fear their partner would not agree to them. However, the sooner you and your partner can uncover all the differences, the sooner you will be able to work with a compromise.

- **Managing stress as a team:** Stress is inevitable in our lives. All that matters are the means that we put into use for handling it. When your partner feels stressed or disturbed, always be by their side as a support. Do not just try to fix all the issues on your own. Allow your partner to work through the issues on their own, in the way they like. Just let your partner be aware of that you are right behind them for providing all the required support. It will provide your partner with a feeling of care and support, the things that matter in a healthy relationship.

- **Offering thanks daily:** It is very beneficial to have a mutual appreciation for one another in a relationship. It is also of prime importance to provide thanks for all the other life aspects. Remember, grateful people are always happy. A couple that feels grateful for having each other can easily build a strong and healthy relationship. No matter what your partner does for you, try to be grateful for that. Be grateful to your life for gifting your partner as constant support. It is the minute things that make our lives beautiful.

- **Be available:** At times, when you need your partner, do you need them to be readily available for you? Or, will you just be able to handle the situation on your own by allowing your partner to prioritize something else before you?

When you wish to be placed first, you will need to start by putting your partner in the first place. Always be ready to help your partner if they need help or you. There is no need to drop all your tasks whimsically. Just be sure of what you will do if your partner needs your support or help suddenly. All your actions during their need hour will help in setting the future tone.

- **Having dinner together:** People tend to bond the most over shared food. So, try to get the most out of it. Plan a romantic dinner. Set up some nice music, dress properly, and connect. That is all it takes. What you are going to eat does not matter. All you need is the full and undivided attention of both of you. Try to talk your heart out, laugh together, and make some good memories. There is no need for any fancy place to bond over dinner. You can set up a nice dinner at your home.
- **Working towards being a better companion:** If you are like all other people, there are certain things that you would like to change regarding yourself. All these desired changes can help in affecting your relationship in a positive way. As you try to be a better person for the sake of your love, you are also trying to be better for yourself.

You are not required to settle. You can aim to develop your relationship and turn it into something that will persistently improve your life. When you are in a strong and happy relationship, it will start resembling all those things that you adore. You will need to concentrate on developing, learning, and continuously having the hope to improve. Remember that it is completely okay to have arguments with your partner. It has been found that all those couples who have arguments can develop better connections. No true relationship will look like a chocolate cake, no flaws, and no arguments. You might think of arguments as a disappointment in your relationship. But, in actuality, they are the building pillars of a strong relationship. As you argue with proper consideration for one another, it will indicate that you are invested in the relationship.

A strong relationship can be developed when two people cooperate with each other for building a life together. A solid relationship can be compared with a trinity; two individuals try to make other things more superior and profound to themselves while being their true selves. To develop a healthy relationship, you will need to develop yourself as an individual and not lose hold of yourself.

Enjoying To Be In Love

Have you fallen in love newly? Then, you must be feeling great at this moment! I have some nice tips for you that can help keep your love strong for a long time and get the most of your new love. To start with it, take enough time and space to enjoy your new love. It indicates that you will have less amount of time for your friend circle. Your true friends will surely understand this and be a part of your happiness. But, do not allow it to be a long trend. You will need to give attention to your friends too. Try to do all those things that you wanted to do for a long. With shared experiences, both of you can be together throughout your relationship. The base of a successful relationship is mainly built of shared experiences. Opt for going out together, watch movies, visit an amusement park, etc.

Make sure you show effort for knowing your partner's friends and ensure that you introduce your partner to your circle of friends. Acceptance in the mutual friend circle can also depict a lot about how two partners can harmonize together. Invite your friends and make sure that they do not feel you both are not paying attention to them. Additionally, serious talks should not be opted out regardless of the prevailing romance. Do not leave a chance to celebrate the shared romance as it can provide you with the strength to fight bad times and sets up common ground. Conversations are of equal importance as experiences. Always share your deep-seated feelings with your partner and provide them the chance to know you well.

Useful Tips For A Happy And Long Relationship

The tips in this section can help you make your relationship happy and strong over time.

- **Stop nagging:** Any form of criticism related to the eccentricities of your partner can result in quarrels. It can also give you an annoying feeling. It has been found that as you try to criticize your partner, you are actually projecting your shortcomings. Instead of making your partner feel frustrated with all your complaints, try to think of how their traits make you feel uncomfortable. Try to reframe your viewpoint about the same. Nagging isn't going to provide you any help or the relationship. You need to look for alternatives or just alter your viewpoint.
- **Accepting the mistakes of your partner:** Human beings make errors. Your romantic partner is not an angel. So, as being human beings, they are bound to make errors or mistakes. When

such things happen, train your mind to forgive. Do not just capitalize on your partner's mistakes. Above everything, there are various things that you cannot change regarding your partner. So, instead of just nagging or grumbling, learn to stay with them. Small mistakes are bound to happen. If you face difficulties in coping with your partner's eccentricities, try to draw their attention to the same. Try to explain your point of view, politely. Do not just focus on accusing or blaming your partner. Opt for simple discussions.

- **Understanding that your partner is a different individual:** You will need to understand that no individual is the same. Your partner is a completely different personality who comes with his/her unique features. However, sometimes, consciously or subconsciously, we try to treat our romantic partner in a way as if they are our extensions. You will need to accept that your partner is a different human being with a unique character that belongs to them. Their perceptions, feelings, experiences, and opinions will not be the same as yours.

- **Not tolerating destructive behavior:** Learn to accept your partner's behaviors until they are not destructive or is life-threatening. If you find that your partner is very aggressive at times, do not just suppress the situation and learn to accept. Nothing is more important than your safety. If you get threatening feelings from your partner, there is no need to stick around them. Just get out of such a relationship. It will be a better choice for both of you.

- **Addressing the problems:** No partnership in this world comes with overall harmony. Both of you are completely different from each other. Your feelings and thoughts are also different. No matter how much dedication or love you both feel for one another, a successful relationship is the result of various compromises. In place of just holding onto long-standing problems, try to discuss the issues directly with your partner. Work together as one team to find the most suitable solution for the problems. Try to interpret problems as a sign of a relationship that is not going to work. As long as you can discuss difficult points, your relationship will last.

Remember that your partner cannot read your mind. You can expect a certain degree of empathy from your partner. However, rely on it completely will result in misunderstandings. So, try to face the difficult matters head-on instead of just waiting for the perfect time. It will be of no help if you keep waiting for your partner to address the issues. Successful communication can help in making your relationship last long and be successful.

- **Taking emotional time out:** Human skin needs exposure to sunlight for getting vitamin D. But frequent and prolonged exposure to long sunlight can result in skin cancer, which can be life-threatening. So, you are required to have an idea of the perfect dosage. The same thing goes for relationships also. Indeed, we will need to fill the lives of one another with happiness. However, we also need to have an idea of emotional time-outs. Taking emotional time-outs indicates not thinking of the other person for some time. You are also required to do something on your own, for your good. Try to determine when is the right time to opt for an emotional break. You can go out with your close friends or just hit a bar and have some fun on your own. You can also opt for solo traveling. Doing so will let you discover and develop yourself as an individual. When both of you can think and experience differently, then only you can have something to discuss at the dinner table.

- **Not tying conditions with gifts:** A gift has to be a gift. In an intimate relationship, it would be unjust if you attach conditions to a favor or gift. If you are willing to do something special for your partner, move ahead without any ulterior motive. Do not play games like, "I will give you a back massage if you also give me the same." The same thing goes for the cost of gifts. Only because you have gifted your partner a diamond ring, that does not mean you can expect a gift of the same value for you. Try to accept favors or gifts in the way they are. They are nothing but symbols and gestures of true love. The same also goes for compliments. We often have the habit of not taking praises and compliments from our partner in a serious way. However, only because your partner loves you, that cannot make their compliments and opinions worthless. If your partner tells you that you are looking pretty, accept that compliment. Do not try to disappoint your partner by saying, "You always say the same thing."

- **Appreciating all those things that you can see in your partner:** The initial infatuation cannot just disappear forever. The majority of the time, it will give ways to other feelings, that of intimate love and attachment. You have discovered that you can depend on your partner completely. You have found that your partner thinks you suit the best for them, and as a couple, you both can harmonize with each other. These are all those things that you have dreamed of always. But as now they have turned into reality, you cannot make up your mind to appreciate them? Try to consider the place of your romantic partner from all these viewpoints. You will come to see how happy you truly are for having them. Show some of that gratitude and happiness to your partner. Talk with your partner regarding how you feel being in love with them.
- **Romantic outings:** The best way to enjoy your closeness is by taking out some time from daily routine and indulging in romantic outings. You can opt for taking a short walk with your partner in the fall or arrange a special movie night in the backyard. Our busy everyday schedule can dull the magic of love between partners. For breaking the monotony, get away from your daily

routine and try to rediscover your relationship. After all, for a strong and healthy relationship, you have to work a lot for it.

The Love Affair Errors

During the periods of fights or emotional turmoil, partners might have irrational thoughts at times that can never help their relationship in any way. Some of such notions are:

- **You always need a partner to be happy:** There are many singles out there who are desperately searching for a partner as they think it is important to have a partner by their side for being happy. If they fail to do so, their life will be less fun and no happiness. Every individual in this world is different from the other. The version of 'happiness' also differs from one person to the other. It is possible to feel good in life even without a partner.
- **Children can be the only savior of a relationship:** It is not at all a good idea to have this notion that having a child can improve a relationship. Indeed, children are wonderful. However, they also tend to put a lot of stress and new challenges on a relationship. If your relationship is

already filled with conflicts, you must think carefully about having a baby. You can wait for some more time so that the number of conflicts can be reduced. Children can only be enriching when their parents know very well that they will get less time to spend with each other. Also, having a child can add up more to financial responsibilities.

- **Dependencies cannot make you happy:** Do not make a mistake and then put all the positive feelings and experiences into your relationship. Always mote that it is you who can make yourself happy in the best way. Do not just hand over the responsibility to your partner. Do not make yourself completely relied on your partner for being happy. Try to preserve your ability to be the responsible one for your happiness and yourself. You will allow your relationship to be more stable and grow easily in this way. Also, both of you can be happier in the relationship, knowing that no one depends on the other.

- **Relationship and sex do not always belong together:** The requirement of having sex in a healthy relationship will vary from one individual to the other. Several couples tend to live their sex life passionately. Some couples get intimate very rarely but are still very romantic. It is important to remember that both partners are required to be equally happy in a relationship with the level of intimacy. A relationship will be successful when both of you can acknowledge the requirements of one another. If you have any problem in this regard, it will be of no help if you shy away from having an open discussion. Only you and your partner will be aware of what is perfect for the relationship. Try to come to a common ground in such cases. If you want to be intimate with your partner more often than your partner, discuss it openly with your partner.

Chapter 11: Everyone Deserves A Wholesome And Healthy Relationship

We all deserve someone who will love you with no conditions. You deserve someone who will not move from their promise to stay with you at times when you are anxious and depressed. You deserve an individual in your life who will not run away when things in the relationship turn out to be difficult. You deserve someone who will not abandon you at times when you require them the most. Always hold out for that person who takes up the delight of treating you in the right way. Hold that person who can provide you with the respect you deserve, meet your required standards, and provide you with proper honesty. A person who deserves all your time is the one who will not just say that they hold strong and genuine feelings for you. They will take the necessary steps to prove their words. Hold someone who can put all their efforts into arranging dates and be romantic with you, someone who can go to any extent for keeping the relationship strong.

An individual who is worth your love is the one who can make you feel loved all the time, not someone who makes you wonder whether their feelings have reduced for you. Natural anxiety is something completely different from the anxiety caused by a partner who is not present. Try to be with a person who will provide their attention to you without asking for it. Be with a person who is not scared of letting the world know how proud they feel to have you. A person who can still love you even after knowing all your flaws is the one that you should treasure. Somebody who can accept that you are the kind of person who overreacts and overthinks and always does what they can do for calming your insecurities is worth keeping.

You deserve unbiased love from a person who is always happy to stay by your side for your entire life. However, you should never take for granted the love you get from your family and friends. You are required to surround yourself with all those who can help bring out the best in you. Keep yourself away from all those you always want to magnify your flaws, tear you down, and make you feel you cannot progress in life. Above all, you need to love yourself. You might overthink, suffer from anxiety, and worry often. But those are not the reasons for disliking who you are. Stop criticizing your flaws; otherwise, you can never stop criticizing others. Do not just that there is something wrong you and changing that will make your life better. You deserve a wholesome relationship and happiness, but you will need to be in love with yourself first.

What Are The Aspects That Can Make A Relationship Healthy?

What is a healthy relationship? There are several factors and qualities behind actions and emotions that help in structuring healthy relationships. All the extra-ordinary romances that can be seen have one thing in common – they result from a commitment to the continued mastery of the relationship skills. Applying all those skills daily is important. The development of patterns and habits for maintaining an extra-ordinary relationship requires an acute form of self-awareness along with the application of excellent communication and behavior.

Developing The Links You Desire

As you keep thinking about what makes a relationship healthy, remember that understanding your partner's desires requires communication. You are not required to be a mind reader. Take to your heart all those things that have been discussed in this relationship book. Learn to discuss with your partner about their wants and needs. After you have successfully recognized the desires of both of you, you can easily work on them to ensure that positive expectations are achieved. Work on the development of your desires, and you will be able to succeed in your relationship.

Trusting Your Partner And Yourself

Trust is always regarded as the foundation stone of a healthy and productive relationship. From trust comes respect. Each of the measures is necessary for interaction, sharing, and relationship growth. It will be during the time of extreme uncertainty and stress when your commitment to mutual nature will be put under doubt. You can find out the extent to which both of you can trust one another. Will your romantic partner trust you for being with them, even at times when you are uncertain or stressed? Will your romantic partner trust you for being clear and honest with them, even when what you might say hurt them? Does your partner trust you to meet all their needs? As you both start trusting each other and yourselves, setting up a healthy relationship is not going to be tough.

Relationships are bound to travel through ups and downs. Sticking by each other even at times of difficulties depicts a healthy and ever-lasting relationship.

Conclusion

Thank you for making it through to the end of the *Book Title*; let's hope it was informative and able to provide you with all of the tools you need to achieve your goals, whatever they may be.

Love is an enjoyable experience when you get rid of your anxieties that tend to come between you and your romantic partner. When you allow anxiety to have a free run in your love life, it might be difficult to determine how and when to react to certain sensitive situations. It will make you feel unconcerned or indifferent to the important issues of your relationship. It might also depict you as being forceful while communicating with your partner. Indeed, it is not your fault. It will be helpful for you if you can understand the effects of anxiety in the way you see things.

Whenever you feel that anxiety is trying to keep you down, you will have to fight it for your relationship and well-being. By taking this book's help and using all the techniques and tips, you can easily overcome all your insecurities and anxieties in your relationship. All the strategies discussed in this book can help you learn positive attitudes for adapting and managing all your anxieties in the right way. Anxiety is the worst enemy of a healthy relationship. It is tough to overcome the same, but it is not impossible.

Finally, if you found this book useful in any way, a review on Amazon is always appreciated!

www.ingramcontent.com/pod-product-compliance
Lightning Source LLC
Chambersburg PA
CBHW071827080526
44589CB00012B/942